D1460934

HOW TO (
SUCCESSFULLY WITH

Awarded for excellence
to Arts & Libraries

Kent
County
Council

Wellhouse Publishing Ltd

First published in Great Britain in 2001 by
Wellhouse Publishing Ltd
31 Middle Bourne Lane
Lower Bourne
Farnham
Surrey GU10 3NH

DISCLAIMER

The aim of this book is to provide general information only and
should not be treated as a substitute for the medical advice of your
doctor or any other health care professional. The publisher and
author is not responsible or liable for any diagnosis made by a
reader based on the contents of this book. Always consult your doctor if you are in any way concerned about your health.

A catalogue record for this book is available from the British Library

ISBN 1 903784 02 6

Printed and bound in Great Britain by
Biddles Ltd., Surrey. www.biddles.co.uk

Contents

Introduction 4

Part I: Diabetes Explained

1 Understanding Diabetes 9
2 People with Diabetes – Some Case Histories 13

Part II: Living with Type 1 Diabetes

3 A Model for Managing Type 1 Diabetes 23
4 Understanding Hyperglycaemia, Ketoacidosis
   and Hypoglycaemia 31
5 Eating Right 41
6 Organizing Your Insulin 53
7 Tests and Targets 59

Part III: Living with Type 2 Diabetes

8 A Global Problem 67
9 Type 2 Diabetes and the Metabolic Syndrome 75
10 Being in Control 81
11 Keeping Glucose Levels Down 87

Part IV: Complications

12 Why You Mustn't Smoke – And How to Stop If You Do 97
13 Keeping Complications at Bay 103
14 'Microvascular' Complications 109
15 'Macrovascular' Complications 113
16 Less Common Problems 117
17 Diabetes in Pregnancy 119
18 Future Treatments 121

Useful Addresses 123
Glossary 124
References 126
Index 127

Introduction

The greatest Olympian of all time and all countries is Britain's oarsman, Sir Steven Redgrave. Anyone who watched the Sydney Olympics knows that he is the first athlete in endurance events ever to win gold medals in five successive Olympics.

He also has diabetes.

If there was ever a role model for people with diabetes, insulin-dependent or otherwise, Sir Steven Redgrave is it. Of course, few people with diabetes can aspire to his athletic heights. But every one of them can take heart from the way he has put his body through the most rigorous training of all, yet still kept good control over his diabetes and remained super-fit.

Rowing is a punishing and gruelling sport. It is a huge feat to keep at the top for more than 16 years, even without diabetes. With it, the task was surely insurmountable. Until now.

That's because we know so much more than we used to about how to control diabetes, and how to keep people with it free from harm, both in the short and long term. Sir Steven has obviously controlled his diabetes to perfection. The main aim of this book is to help others to emulate him – not in a search for Olympic gold, but at least in achieving the quality of life he so obviously enjoys, despite his health 'hiccup'.

This health 'hiccup' is what most people with diabetes have. Kept under good control, it cannot be looked upon truly as an illness. Today's treatments and management schemes for diabetes have turned it from a fatal disease into an inconvenience that, with sensible control, can be lived with into a normal old age.

This book does not aim to guide potential Sir Steven Redgraves to Olympic medals. But it could do so. Because the rules for diabetes affect everyone who has it, whether it started in childhood or in middle age, whether insulin is needed or not, and whether they are athletes or just average everyday people. What this book does aim to do is to set out the rules. It describes the problems and pitfalls for people with diabetes and their families and carers, and how these issues can be faced and avoided.

Told for the first time they have diabetes, many people feel that they face a life-sentence of poor health and early death. It can be a very unhappy time for children and their parents, and for the adults who, perhaps, until the diagnosis were sailing on through life, unaware of the time-bomb of troubles waiting to blow up in their faces.

Given the example of people like Sir Steven, people told they have diabetes can take a deep breath, put aside their fears, and look forward to a good and long life, just as enjoyable as everyone else's.

This does not mean that people with diabetes can live just like anyone without it. They obviously can't. They must stick closely to the correct healthy eating habits, they must take the correct amount of exercise, and they must comply with their medical team's advice on treatment, be it on insulin or glucose-lowering pills, or high blood pressure lowering drugs. It is a bit harder to be a child, teenager or adult with diabetes than one without it, but facing the challenge is worth the effort.

In fact, there is no alternative. Failing to face up to the challenge can lead to severe health problems. Teenagers who rebel against their fairly strict routine (unhappily a very common occurrence) are courting early blindness, kidney failure, heart attacks, strokes and circulation problems in their limbs. Adults with later-onset diabetes can expect the same problems a few decades later if they don't manage to control their weight, their smoking habits and their blood pressure.

The good news is that good control of diabetes and blood pressure in both children and adults, along with a healthy lifestyle, can greatly extend their length and quality of life, usually well into old age.

So this book describes all aspects of the healthy lifestyle that every person with diabetes needs to follow. It is positive and optimistic: it is more about 'dos' than 'don'ts'. It is full of hope for the future: one chapter deals with the possibility of cure using modern transplant technology. The main purpose of this book, however, is to give people with diabetes a sense that they can shape their own future.

Part One
Diabetes Explained

Chapter One

Understanding Diabetes

Diabetes, it does not need to be said, is a complex subject. Its full title is *diabetes mellitus. Diabetes* is ancient Greek for 'syphon', or a constant flow of water, and *mellitus* is from the Latin word for 'honey'. The two words describe the two main symptoms of the illness: syphon refers to the constant need to drink water and pass urine, both in excess; honey refers to the sweet, honey-like taste of the urine, which is full of sugar – or to be more accurate, glucose. How did the doctors of old know this? In the past they made the diagnosis by tasting their patients' urine. Happily, 21st-century doctors do not have to do the same!

Diabetes mellitus is in fact two different diseases. One starts usually in childhood, is caused by failure of the pancreas to produce insulin, and needs daily insulin injections. It is defined by doctors as Type 1 diabetes, childhood-onset diabetes, and insulin-dependent diabetes mellitus (or IDDM). The other kind, which usually starts in adulthood, is caused by the build-up in the body's tissues and organs of resistance to the action of insulin. It is called Type 2 diabetes, adult-onset diabetes, and non-insulin-dependent diabetes (or NIDDM). People with Type 2 are still able to produce insulin, and can be treated largely by diet and, if necessary, by oral drugs.

However, in both types of diabetes the general advice on lifestyle is similar, and the long-term complications are roughly the same. Both kinds of diabetes lead to higher risks of strokes and heart attacks, circulation problems, kidney failure and blindness. So, although in this book each type of diabetes has been allocated separate sections covering its origins and specific aspects of tests and treatment, other chapters contain information that is equally applicable and relevant to readers with either type of diabetes.

What is it that makes it essential for people with diabetes to follow such a strict lifestyle? To answer this question we must understand some basic facts about the disease.

Glucose in the Body

The first essential is to understand the importance of glucose in the body. Glucose is the fuel that every cell in our body uses for its energy. We get it from the digestion of starches (mainly from bread, pasta, potatoes and rice) and sugars (mainly from fruit and sweets) in our food. All starches and sugars must be converted to glucose in the small intestine before we can take it up in the bloodstream to circulate around the body. Every cell in the body, no matter where or whatever its function, uses glucose as its basis for energy, and therefore for life. Without glucose, the cell would die.

When we eat meals or drink liquids that contain starches and sugars, within a few minutes (in the case of sugary drinks) or after a longer time (in the case of starches), glucose levels start to rise in the blood. Technically this is described as a rising blood glucose. The glucose has then to be transferred across the walls of the smallest blood vessels (the capillaries) into the tissues. With this transfer, the blood glucose level starts to fall until we next eat or drink.

Once in the cells, the glucose is 'burned' by oxygen to release energy which the cells can then use for all their functions, including the important one of staying alive. Oxygen arrives in the cells via the red blood cells, which pick it up in the lungs (from the air we breathe) and carry it through the heart and around the body to the capillaries. There the red cells give up the oxygen to be transferred through the capillary walls into the tissues, where it can reach the cells.

The whole process of burning glucose with oxygen could be compared with what happens in an internal combustion engine. In the cylinder, a spark of oxygen from the air intake causes a droplet of petrol to explode, providing the energy for the engine to run. In our human machine we use the same oxygen, but this time the fuel is glucose rather than petrol. Glucose is 'burned', releasing energy for the cells to use and then finishing up as carbon dioxide and water, which we excrete through our lungs and kidneys, which act much like the exhaust pipes in a car.

The Role of Insulin

Glucose cannot reach the tissues on its own, however. We need insulin in the bloodstream to 'drive' the glucose from the blood across the capillary walls into the tissues. So, shortly after eating or drinking sugary or starchy foods, not only does the blood glucose rise, but blood insulin levels rise, too. The pancreas, the organ that makes insulin, detects and responds to rising blood glucose levels by injecting insulin into the blood. As the blood insulin level rises, it drives the excess glucose into the tissues, where most of it is used to provide energy for the cells to perform their functions.

Such functions could be the contraction of a muscle, a thought in the brain, the reception of light in the eye, a chemical process in the liver, or the filtering of waste from the blood by a kidney cell. All these functions need glucose and oxygen, and insulin is necessary to get the glucose to the crucial spot.

One of our design 'faults' as human beings is that we cannot store glucose in our cells. So for our bodies to keep active we need a constant supply of fresh glucose to our muscles, brain, heart and all our other organs. We therefore must keep our blood glucose levels at the correct level, so that we never run short of our fuel. A car stops when the petrol flow to the cylinder fails. The same applies to a failure of glucose delivery to our cells – we shut down. Too low a blood glucose level and we become 'hypoglycaemic' (hypo = under; glyc = glucose; aemic = relating to 'haem' or blood). A hypoglycaemic brain (a brain through which the flowing blood contains too little glucose) shuts down its activity to conserve energy – and we lose consciousness. But too high a blood glucose level (hyperglycaemia) may have the same result – because the mechanism that transfers glucose out of the capillaries and into the tissues (i.e. insulin) has failed.

This is where diabetes comes in. Without enough insulin (as in Type 1 diabetes), or when the insulin mechanism fails to shift the glucose out of the blood and into the tissues (as in Type 2 diabetes), blood glucose levels rise because the necessary glucose cannot reach the cells.

In essence, therefore, diabetes is simple to understand. We depend on a constant delivery of glucose to all our tissues for them to act normally and for us to survive. Insulin is the mechanism for doing precisely this – it could be compared with the fuel pump in a car. When the fuel pump goes wrong, no matter how much petrol we have in the tank, it can't reach the cylinder and the vital spark. Without a normal insulin mechanism, the glucose in our bloodstream can't reach the cells.

Glycogen

To complete the picture, we must add a little about the muscles and the liver. Glucose can be stored in both of these organs, but not as glucose itself. For storage, it must be converted into a more complex sugar, glycogen. Then, when we start to call on our immediate energy reserves – say when we are running or starving – we convert the glycogen back into glucose.

Muscles working at their limit convert stored glycogen into glucose and use it immediately. We surely have all experienced a 'stitch': this is the pain we get when we have used up all the glycogen in our muscles and we start to run on 'empty'. The muscle uses fats instead, and that causes a build-up of lactic acid inside them. The acid causes the typical pain of a stitch. More than that, when fats are used instead of glucose for energy purposes, they do not break down as glucose does into carbon dioxide and water, but into 'ketones'. These are released in the urine, and sometimes in the breath. We will have much more to say about ketones later.

The liver's glycogen stores are also a back-stop against starvation and excessive exercise. Once the circulating glucose in the blood starts to fall below a critical level, the liver, like the muscles, converts stored glycogen into glucose and pushes it out into the bloodstream, from which the tissues can suck it out and use it.

So the normal person has two ways of providing glucose for the cells. One is directly via the glucose in the bloodstream from the food and drink we digest. The second is from the glycogen stores from the liver and the muscles.

The crucial thing to understand about both these processes is that they are wholly dependent on a normal insulin system. It is insulin that stimulates the release by the liver of glucose from its glycogen stores, and it is insulin that stimulates the conversion of glycogen into glucose inside the muscles.

So people with diabetes of either type have two major problems. They not only cannot get their circulating glucose into their cells, but they also cannot convert their glycogen stores into much needed glucose at times of high energy need.

Just think of coping with these two problems when you are an Olympic athlete, pushing your muscles to the normal limit and beyond, and marvel at Sir Steven Redgrave's accomplishment! If he can get his insulin dose right to control his supply of glucose to his muscles and to manage his glycogen stores, both to perfection, how much simpler it must be for most ordinary people, with ordinary problems, to manage theirs!

Chapter Two

People with Diabetes – Some Case Histories

The explanation of diabetes as outlined in Chapter One is probably better understood by presenting some case histories. If you have diabetes yourself, or are reading this to know more about a relative's diabetes, then you will surely recognize one of the following descriptions.

Jamie

Jamie was 8 years old when he fell ill. Previously a healthy little boy, doing well at school, the change in his health was dramatic. He was always thirsty, needing to drink far more often, and far more, than his brothers and sisters and his classmates. He was also visiting the toilet far more often, to pass urine – a fact that his teacher noticed (because it disturbed his class) before his mother did (because he was quietly slipping off on his own at home to do it). He retained his healthy appetite, yet he was losing weight, becoming noticeably thinner over only a week or two.

Most worrying of all, Jamie did not feel well. He had vague muscle pains, had a constant ache in his back, especially before passing urine, and he felt weak and tired. He could no longer keep up with his classmates in the school playground: from being a leader in games he became a watcher. His school work was suffering, too, in that he was sleepier than usual during the day, and could not concentrate.

His teacher brought her worries about him to his mother, whose fears that he was ill were then confirmed. A rapid visit to the doctor led to a fast diagnosis, and admission to the local children's ward for initial control of his Type 1 diabetes and the start of his long-term self-management.

Now 45, Jamie remembers the day he started on insulin as if it were yesterday. In his student years he played soccer for his university. He passed through the rigorous training as a medical student with relative ease, and without any health problems. A doctor now, he keeps his diabetes under tight control, and has reaped the benefit of doing so, with a happy and healthy family life and, so far, no complications. He helps hundreds of other people with diabetes in his large hospital diabetes clinic. He is a great example for them to follow.

Jenny

In complete contrast to Jamie's case, Jenny didn't notice anything wrong until she was in her mid-40s. Even then, she assumed that her troubles were due to her approaching middle age and menopause. Her main worry was that she had put on weight – about 2 stone (13 kg) over the past few months. She also felt less 'energetic', tending to drop off to sleep in the early evenings, and not feeling much like going out and doing things. She also admitted to being 'a bit thirsty' and, for the first time in her life, needing to get up once or twice every night to pass urine.

More embarrassingly, she complained of an itch around, and a discharge from, her vagina. This, too, was a first for her. It had been a source of worry for her and her husband, who also had an itch. Happily, neither blamed the other for the problem.

Her doctor found large amounts of glucose in her urine, and confirmed her Type 2 diabetes by performing a blood glucose test on the spot. The doctor gently explained that Jenny had Type 2 diabetes and, after giving her some reassurance, arranged for Jenny and her husband to come back later that day. At that meeting the doctor gave them the time they needed to learn much more about the illness and how they could cope with it. Jenny and her husband were also given immediate treatment for her thrush infection, a common cause of genital itch in newly diagnosed or difficult-to-control diabetes.

The practice team was told about the new case of diabetes, and Jenny was added to the diabetes clinic list. In modern medical practice, Type 2 diabetes is managed by the primary care team of general practitioner, specialized diabetes nurse and dietician. Jenny met all of them at her next visit a few days later.

Alec

Alec is 45 and a busy newspaperman. An ex-soccer player, he is less fit than he was. He spends a lot of his time at a computer keyboard, and has put a little around his middle in the last few years. But that isn't why he came to his doctor.

He had an itchy foreskin, and it sometimes 'burnt' a little when he passed urine. It looked red and occasionally there was a small bead of pus at the end of the opening of the foreskin. He is a happily married family man, and he knew that he had not 'strayed', so that it was very unlikely to be a sexually transmitted disease. But from what he had read in magazines, it seemed very much like one.

Only after several weeks of applying creams and taking herbal preparations did he pluck up enough courage to see his doctor – who immediately put his mind at rest.

Alec had thrush, or to give it its medical name, an infection with the germ candida albicans. A microscopic fungus, rather than a bacterium or virus, thrush, like yeast, thrives on sugar. That was the clue to the diagnosis. Thrush infections in the penis in men are often the only sign of a new case of diabetes – and his doctor was quick to test the urine for glucose. It was full of it.

A blood test confirmed the diagnosis. Alec was astounded by the news. He had not had the slightest idea that he might have diabetes. He wasn't particularly thirsty, nor had he been passing, for him, an excessive amount of urine. Though once he had started on the correct diet and began exercising again, losing the excess weight in the process, he realised that he had been under par. He felt more energetic, less tired, and less lethargic, especially in the evenings after his last meal of the day. He had thought that his tiredness had just been a part of his general unfitness. He now understands that it was the onset of his Type 2 diabetes.

Alec is now back to fitness training on four evenings a week. He is back to his match weight, and is managing his diabetes on diet alone. However, he still attends the diabetic clinic at his local health centre once a month, just to make sure that he is in control.

How did he catch his thrush infection? Thrush organisms are normal inhabitants of most people's bowel, where most of the time they are almost completely suppressed by the rest of the normal bowel germs. He may have unwittingly spread thrush germs from the skin around the anus forward to the penis in something as mundane as his bath water. The sugar in microscopic spots of urine under the foreskin did the rest. So there is no need for embarrassment or blame – and certainly no need to be guilty about a possible transmissible disease. Now that he has no glucose in his urine he no longer has thrush infections.

Mary

Mary became pregnant for the first time at 31, she and her husband having decided to put off having a family until they could afford it – a fairly common decision these days. So she was very upset when, at her second antenatal visit when around 12 weeks pregnant, her routine urine sample showed a moderate amount of glucose. She had been feeling well, and so the news shocked her. Knowing a little about diabetes because an aunt had had it, she was fearful that her baby might be affected, and that she might fall ill during the pregnancy.

The antenatal team was able to reassure her. A 'fasting blood glucose level' was taken the next morning. This was a glucose measurement from blood taken before breakfast after a light meal 12 hours before. It showed a glucose level a little higher than normal, a sign that Mary did have diabetes, but not necessarily a kind that would last beyond her pregnancy.

The next step was for her to have an 'oral glucose tolerance test' or OGTT. For this she was asked to swallow 50 grams of glucose; her blood glucose levels were measured just before doing so, then at regular intervals for a few hours afterwards. The OGTT showed that her blood glucose rose higher than normal and stayed there, only returning towards the normal level very slowly.

Mary was then sent to a diabetes team specializing in diabetes during pregnancy – known as 'gestational diabetes' – where she was given advice on a healthy diet and on how to lose weight (she was more than 2 stone overweight). She was taught how to measure her own blood glucose level, and was not given anti-diabetes drugs.

For the rest of her pregnancy Mary was watched for any rise in glucose levels. Happily, she took to the diet well, lost some weight, and her blood glucose levels remained under the crucial levels of 6 millimoles per litre (mmol/L) before meals and 9 millimoles per litre after meals. *There is more in later chapters on these measurements.* If levels had gone above these thresholds, she would have been given insulin.

Mary's pregnancy was a great success. She had a healthy baby boy weighing just over 8 pounds. Six weeks afterwards, at the routine post-natal visit to her doctor, her blood glucose level was back to normal. However, she is not necessarily cured of her diabetes. About 40 per cent of women like Mary with gestational diabetes go on in later life to develop Type 2 diabetes. She was warned of this fact, and has been asked to keep up her new lifestyle, with the correct eating habits, regular exercise and weight control. She has been healthy now for 10 years. She runs, walks, cycles and swims with her 10-year old son and her admiring husband, and has every chance of avoiding diabetes if she continues as she has done so far.

Derek

Derek's story is not so hopeful. A heavy drinker since his teens, at 45 he started to feel decidedly unwell. His hangovers were lasting longer than the next morning. He felt sick most of the next day, and tended to take the 'hair of the dog' in the early evening to help himself feel better. This did not work.

What eventually brought Derek to his doctor was a constant pain right across the small of his back. It was so bad that he used a hot-water bottle to ease the pain, and in doing so burned himself, leaving the skin red and blistered.

By this time he had lost a lot of weight, and his appetite. He did not directly complain of thirst, but as he was in the habit of consuming large quantities of beer most days, a change in his fluid consumption and urine output might have been difficult to spot.

What his doctor did not find difficult to spot was that Derek looked ill and faintly jaundiced. His stomach was slightly swollen, and he was very tender when the doctor pressed a hand on his abdomen, just below the bottom of his breastbone.

Blood tests showed that Derek had chronic pancreatitis, a condition very common in heavy drinkers. He needed to be taken off all alcohol, and was brought into hospital to try to reverse the damage and to see if the liver, too, was affected. During the extensive hospital tests, Derek was found to have diabetes. Unlike the others described above, his diabetes was a direct result of the damage that alcohol had caused to his pancreas, which could no longer make enough insulin for his needs. In effect, he had a form of Type 1 diabetes, even though it had started when he was an adult.

Derek was told by his doctors that alcohol was now a virtual poison for him, and that his only hope of future health was to become teetotal and to follow the strict diet and exercise rules that all people with Type 1 diabetes must follow. He did that for several years, but eventually he failed to come to his regular follow-up appointments and it was heard indirectly that he had started drinking again. In this case his health will deteriorate very quickly.

Sadru

Sadru was 43 when he attended a doctor for a routine medical for life assurance, organized by his employers. He was astonished when he was refused, and was asked to see his own doctor for a check up. Because life assurance doctors act for the insurers, and not for the 'insuree', he was not given any details about why he had been refused.

His own doctor, who had not seen him for years, picked up two solid reasons for the insurance company's refusal to cover Sadru. One was high blood pressure, the other was glucose in his urine ('glycosuria'). Sadru's first reaction to these test results was disbelief. Why, if he was so ill, he asked, did he not feel unwell? His doctor went over the last few years of Sadru's life in detail. Was he still doing the things he was doing five years ago, for example? Well, no, was the reply. He was no longer taking so much exercise. He had been promoted into a much more responsible job. It meant business dinners, late nights, many stressful decisions to make, and more time at his desk, in the car and on planes. He had put on 2 stone in weight, mostly around his middle. No, he had not noticed if he was less fit than before, but that was mainly because he could not remember when he had last had enough physical exercise to make him breathless.

It turned out, when he had a fitness check on a treadmill with a cardiac monitor strapped to his chest, that Sadru was decidedly less fit than he thought. Not only was his OGTT verging towards diabetes, he had a high blood cholesterol level, and high insulin levels, too.

His doctor diagnosed 'syndrome X': a combination of high blood pressure, high cholesterol level, high blood glucose and 'central obesity' (meaning that he was apple-shaped, with his main fat around his stomach, rather than pear-shaped, with the main fat around his buttocks and hips). This combination of problems is very well known to doctors, especially in people, like Sadru, whose parents originated from the Indian subcontinent. It is entirely due to the insulin resistance mentioned in the previous chapter. It needs very strict treatment to avoid an early death due to a heart attack or stroke. Which is why Sadru had been refused his life assurance.

To give Sadru credit, once his position had been made clear to him he made some very important decisions about his life. He made sure he took time to 'stop and smell the roses'. More quality time with his family, more exercise, far better eating habits, and learning to relax have made all the difference. Over the last five years he has lost the extra weight, his blood pressure has fallen to normal levels, there is no glucose in his urine, and his blood glucose levels (including his OGTT) have returned to within normal limits. His cholesterol level was more difficult to control, but it has eventually fallen on a 'statin' drug – about which more later. After all this time, a life assurance company has given Sadru a policy that recognizes he now has a future. But this is no cure. His syndrome X is under control, but it will come back if he returns to his former habits. He is determined not to do so.

Tom

Then there's me. When I was 29, in rural general practice, I caught the mumps. It surprised me, because I had looked after many children with this infection without any thought that I might not have had it myself as a child. Obviously I hadn't. I woke one morning with what appeared to be a rugby ball broadside in my throat, and made my own diagnosis with a brief look in the mirror.

I was relatively lucky, in that I didn't develop the one complication that most men dread – inflammation of the testes (orchitis). But I did have a niggling pain in the centre of the upper abdomen, just under the ribs, which lasted the same amount of time as the swollen glands in my neck. It wasn't a bad pain, and didn't stop me working. I continued to see patients who had had mumps, which tends to suggest that my illness was minor.

Four years later, having put on a little weight, I wasn't feeling too well. I'm 5 foot 10 and my usual weight is 12 stone (76 kilograms). At 33 I had changed my job. Now in a research post, I spent far more time sitting, much less time walking, and had given up my running and football training. I had slowly gained 2 stone (13 kilograms), almost without noticing. I was sleepy in the evenings, hadn't my usual energy even to mow the lawn, and was getting a bit short-tempered with my long-suffering wife and two small children.

It was my wife, who has no medical or nursing training, who suggested that I might have diabetes. I laughed at the preposterous suggestion, but I took a urine sample just the same. It contained glucose. So I know how it feels to be labelled as 'diabetic' – an excellent lesson for any doctor. I'm firmly of the belief that every doctor should have a similar experience, just to know what it is like to be on the other end of the stethoscope.

I was lucky. All I had to do was lose weight, start exercising again and eat healthily. My OGTT, which had been verging on the diabetic, returned to normal. It seems that the abdominal pain I had had with the mumps was a mild pancreatitis, and that it had reduced my capacity to produce insulin. So long as I don't put too great a load on my pancreas, it will produce enough insulin for all normal needs.

How do I go about this? From the day of my diagnosis I resolved to change my tastes. It was far easier than I thought. No more sugar in tea and coffee. No more sugar-filled desserts. My sources of carbohydrates from then on were bread, pasta, rice and potatoes, plus fresh fruit. I never eat more than I need, and often rise from the table still feeling a little hungry. Even now, many years later, I feel hungry most of the time. I find that a little exercise every day curbs this appetite.

I started running again, and felt better within a few days. Within two months I had lost nearly 2 stone (13 kg). My OGTT was normal, and it has remained normal ever since. I no longer have glucose in my urine, and my fasting blood glucose is around 3 to 4 mmol/L. I feel fine, but do not let my weight rise above 13 stone (82 kg).

Helping Yourself

These case histories have been chosen because they are typical of the range of people who develop diabetes as children or adults. You may find your own history, or something close to it, among them. The chapters that follow use these people's stories to illustrate how diabetes is managed and the problems and pitfalls that may affect people like them.

The aim in every case is not just to keep people relatively well. Probably the most apt quote on the treatment of diabetes was by Professor Robert Tattersall, a much-respected British diabetes specialist and researcher. 'Diabetes', he wrote, 'is an easy disease to treat badly'. The aim of the next few chapters is to make sure that you treat yourself well. Because you are the main person in your treatment. Others can only give advice. You are the only person who can put that advice into practice.

If your diabetes is badly treated, you may still avoid the immediate problems of comas and 'hypos' – about which more later. But you will be laying yourself open to serious complications over the next 20 years or so – such as a heart attack, stroke, blindness, kidney failure and gangrene of the limbs. We know now that good blood glucose control and good blood pressure control – the two go hand in hand in diabetes – will greatly help to prevent them all. The next few chapters put these risks into context and spell out exactly why you should be strict with yourself, so that you can avoid them.

Part Two
Living with Type 1 Diabetes

Chapter Three

A Model for Managing
Type 1 Diabetes

Jamie's diagnosis was made more than 30 years ago, when he was 8 years old. At that time, the main aim of managing diabetes in children was to control their diabetes so that they were able to live a reasonably normal life. The emphasis then was on three essentials – eating correctly, exercising, and keeping their insulin injections in tune with their food intake and their exercise levels.

Children around Jamie's age with diabetes were taught to give their own insulin injections, and how to recognize when things were getting out of control. They had to know themselves when they were 'hypo' or 'hyper', and how to treat either state. But as long as they kept reasonably in good glucose balance, their doctors felt satisfied that they were doing well.

Nowadays we know this is not nearly enough, either for children or adults with Type 1 diabetes. Today's aim is not just to avoid the unpleasant symptoms of disturbed glucose levels, but to try to keep the blood glucose pattern throughout the whole 24 hours in every day as close to normal as possible. It is easy to keep the glucose levels within a broad band so that you feel relatively well and have no acute problems, but we now recognize that this is not enough. If we wish to do as much as we can to ward off the later complications such as kidney failure, heart attack, stroke and blindness, we need to do much more.

So today, people with Type 1 diabetes must place much more emphasis than ever before on eating healthily, on regular exercise (particularly to keep their weight normal) and on the timing and the doses of their insulin. They must also have regular checks on blood glucose levels, on blood pressure, and on their eyes, kidneys and nervous system.

Luckily Jamie's parents had the foresight to make sure that he understood the importance of good diabetes control. This he knew at primary school. They also recognized that the danger time was in adolescence, and took special care to ensure that he passed through this turbulent phase as easily as possible. Jamie was fortunate in that, wanting to become a doctor, he was particularly interested in the illness and its complications. His teenage years were spent mainly in studying and in trying to make the county's athletics team. His career choice and lei-sure preferences kept him on the straight and narrow, although he would admit now, looking back, that there were times when he could so easily have gone wrong.

Getting the Control Right

The first priority in all types of diabetes is to get the control right. This can only be done by co-ordinating as finely as possible three things – your intake of food, your physical activity, and your dose and type of insulin. You must check yourself whether you are getting it right by reg-ular blood glucose tests, and your doctor or diabetes nurse will double-check by performing an HbA1c test.

HbA1c is a measure of how well you have been controlling your blood glucose levels over the previous 2-3 months.

The principle of the HbA1c test is fairly easy to understand. With glu-cose floating about in the bloodstream all the time, some of it 'sticks' to the haemoglobin, the red pigment inside the red blood cells that carries oxygen around the body. This is known as 'glycosylated haemoglobin' or HbA1c. Only around 4 per cent of the red cells are glycosylated in peo-ple without diabetes: this is read as an HbA1c of 4 per cent. The normal range is taken as between 3 and 6.5 per cent.

In poorly controlled diabetes, in people whose blood glucose levels have been well above normal for many weeks on end, HbA1c can be above 20 per cent. Many people with reasonable control of their dia-betes have HbA1c levels under 8 per cent.

This is important, because it has been proved time and again that lowering the HbA1c lowers the risk of later complications in the eyes, kidneys, nervous system and blood vessels. The risk of all of them rises substantially as the HbA1c climbs above 8 per cent.

The Danish Model

Keeping the HbA1c low isn't simply a matter of getting the food, exer-cise and insulin about right. Particularly for children, it means atten-tion by several different professionals. Even in a sophisticated country like Denmark, as recently as 1997 diabetes centres specializing in children were reporting average HbA1c levels of 9.4 per cent. The Danish specialists in childhood diabetes, shocked by their poor per-formance, therefore decided to reorganize the work of all the medical and paramedical staff to try to improve things. What follows is a model for the management of all Type 1 diabetes, not just for children, but for adults, too.

The first step was to establish a single centre for children's diabetes for Copenhagen. In October 2000 the staff were looking after 203 children. With around 33 new cases per year, within 5 years they will have between 250 and 300 children in their care, 30 per cent of them under school age.

The staff recognized that, despite technical improvements like better ways of measuring blood glucose at home, regular HbA1c tests, better ways of delivering the insulin (mainly with pens – see later), and more choice of insulins, in fact over the previous decade they had not improved the children's diabetes control.

What they needed to do was to increase the children's self-confidence and self-sufficiency, so that they could better come to terms with their diabetes and how to control it.

They had to involve the whole family and inform them about diabetes, and improve their knowledge and skills. They had to attend to the special needs of ethnic minorities with language problems, and of those with learning difficulties. They had to bring the families into the management plans and adapt them to their circumstances. They used the children's own experiences to help treat and provide support for newly diagnosed children.

It meant a lot of work and time, but it succeeded. All the children were treated as outpatients. Diabetes nurse specialists were employed, and weekly meetings of the whole diabetes team were held to discuss problems in specific families coming to the clinic. Families had a 24-hour dedicated hotline to ring in case of any problems. A children's psychologist was brought in, and the staff were given extra education in diabetes management.

The regular team now consists of two specialist physicians in childhood diabetes, three children's general physicians, two specialist nurses, a dietician, a chiropodist, a lab technician, a social worker and a psychologist.

This team laid down the following aims for the children:
● to achieve normal growth and development
● to achieve normal schooling and career goals
● to achieve the optimum quality of life
● to understand about diabetes treatment appropriate to their age

- to keep numbers of complications of diabetes that can affect children (such as eye, kidney and nerve problems) as low as possible
- to train the children to take over their own management at the appropriate age for them
- to transfer them to an adult clinic at the appropriate time

By the time they reach adulthood, the children are very well equipped to care for their own diabetes for the rest of their lives.

The system involves much more attention to detail than before. At 9 years old, every child has three very important examinations: of their eyes, their kidneys, and their nervous system. Their eyes are examined by a specialist ophthalmologist for the earliest evidence of 'diabetic retinopathy', the condition which in the past has led to blindness in so many people with Type 1 diabetes.

The kidney test involves each child having two overnight samples of urine examined for 'microalbuminuria' – tiny amounts of protein in the urine which predict later diabetic kidney disease.

They also have their nervous system examined for loss of the ability to detect vibration against the skin of the feet. This predicts later diabetic neuropathy (in which there is loss of sensation in the limbs, and which can be the first stage in the pathway towards serious damage to the feet).

If the test results are normal and the HbA1c is under 8 per cent, then the child is screened again at age 11, and once a year thereafter. If the test results are not favourable, then the children are seen much more often, and every effort is made, with better control, to return them to normal.

How has the Danish clinic improved the children's control over their diabetes? Both the children and their parents are encouraged to measure blood glucose levels at home much more often than before, and to adjust the insulin dose, diet and physical activity according to the results. The diabetes nurses visit far more often than before – in the first 6 months at least twice a month, then every 2 to 3 months after establishing good control. The dietician, social worker and psychologist also visit as required. Every child has a blood glucose meter, and the results are read by a computer programme – this makes it much easier to adjust the treatment. Children of similar ages and their parents are encouraged to meet regularly to swap information and to be taught new and practical techniques. These sessions are very well attended.

Puberty – The Problem Years

Puberty is a problem for most people, whether or not they have diabetes. It is particularly hard for children with diabetes. The rush of sex hormones, their changing energy needs (from excessive to slothful) and their rapid growth, allied to increased emotional and social pressures, make good control very difficult. The teenager with diabetes going out with friends to parties must still strictly control his or her behaviour in a way that seems unfair, and he or she can often resent it. Only too often they can let themselves go, and that, sadly, can lead to permanent damage to the eyes, kidneys and nerves.

So the teenager with diabetes must have a special counsellor who knows the problems, not just of diabetes but of teenagers, too. Such counsellors are pretty rare, but the Danes have concentrated on finding and training them. They communicate with adolescents on their own terms and negotiate realistic targets of control that their patients can accept. Teenagers with Type 1 diabetes in Copenhagen attend after-school meetings arranged by the specialist nurses and dieticians. They discuss diet, alcohol, how to cope with parties, contraception, worries about pregnancy and childbirth – in fact, all the things that other teenagers need advice on, but rarely get.

Because continuity of care throughout the teenage years is so vital, young adults with diabetes do not leave the children's diabetes system in Denmark until they are 18 – three years after children's hospitals normally pass on their patients to adult clinics. Before the final transfer there are three or more years of overlap, so that the adult team has got to know the patient while still under the children's team's care. This is vital, because it ensures continuity and builds trust in the new team. During the year of transfer, all the teenagers being transferred in that year meet informally together, consolidating that trust and learning about the way the new medical team will continue to help them.

By the time they have reached the adult clinic, all the children who have gone through the Copenhagen scheme have become expert in their own care. They have gone through education schemes prepared jointly by the hospital, schoolteachers and psychologists. They possess information sheets and guidelines on coping with diabetes, and are tested on their knowledge of their diabetes, so that they can be retrained if it is found wanting. Parents and grandparents, school friends and teaching personnel in further education institutes are all included in this education process.

Hitting the Targets

Did the Danish team hit their targets? They were difficult ones to achieve. Where children had HbA1cs of 10 per cent or above, they aimed to lower them to 9 per cent within a year. They aimed at HbA1cs for the children under 6 to be below 9 per cent, and for those aged 7 to 18 years to be below 8.5 per cent in the first two years of diagnosis, and for all children to have HbA1cs under 8 per cent within 4 years.

One reason for the higher (less strict) HbA1c target for the younger children was to avoid bringing the glucose level too low, and thereby causing the occasional severe hypoglycaemic attack, defined as a bout of unconsciousness and convulsions (fits). Such attacks in young children may cause brain damage, leading later to a lower intellect and psychological problems. The clinic's aim was to keep the frequency of these episodes to below 20 for every 100 patients treated for a year. They far exceeded this aim, with no 'hypos' in the younger children and only 3 in the older ones. They reduced the average HbA1c, even of the younger children, to 8 per cent.

Ketosis Attacks

Another aim was to avoid repeated attacks of 'ketosis'. 'Hypo' attacks are the result of the child receiving too much insulin for the amount of glucose circulating in the blood. This can happen when either the insulin dose is too high, or not enough food is eaten after the injection. Ketosis is the opposite: if there is too little insulin in the circulation, the body must use fats rather than glucose for its energy source.

Unlike glucose, which breaks down into carbon dioxide and water when releasing its energy, fats break down into ketones, acid-like chemicals which appear in the breath and the urine, and for which there are simple urine tests. Ketones smell sweet, somewhat like pear drops, so they can be very obvious to people who can smell them (a substantial proportion of the population, including myself, can't). Ketosis is a sign that the person is on the way to a diabetic coma, and should be corrected as soon as possible. This is best done by giving insulin and extra fluids.

A Great Success

The Danish team was highly successful in all their aims. The average HbA1c level in all their children fell from over 9 per cent to 8 per cent. The fall in the teenagers was even greater, from well over 10 per cent to around 7 per cent. Hypo attacks were almost eradicated in doing so – a considerable achievement, as the lower the HbA1c becomes, the greater the chance that on some days the blood glucose may dip and bring on a 'hypo'. And there were no children with repeated attacks of ketosis.

Why have I spent so long on these Danish results? Because they are an example of the best type of diabetes care. Their systems of education, care and follow-up are a model for every group involved in diabetes. If you feel that the care you or your children are receiving falls short of this standard, you should seriously consider why, and talk to your medical team about it. It is long past the time that diabetes was simply a matter of keeping free of 'hypos' and ketosis. That is the easy part. The difficult part is how to keep healthy and free of diabetes-related illness in your future. Before I go into how you can do that, however, there are practical points to consider about day-to-day management of your insulin treatment and of the tests that ensure you are getting things right.

Chapter Four

Understanding Hyperglycaemia, Ketoacidosis and Hypoglycaemia

When you are newly diagnosed with Type 1 diabetes, the first priority is to recognize how it feels to have hyperglycaemic and hypoglycaemic ('hypo') attacks, and to know precisely what to do when they start.

Hyperglycaemia

Hyperglycaemia is uncontrolled diabetes. That is, your blood glucose is too high, mainly because you do not have enough circulating insulin to drive the glucose from the blood into the tissues, so that it cannot be used for all your energy purposes.

One problem with hyperglycaemia is that when the glucose is only moderately raised, you may notice nothing wrong at first. It is only when it persists and becomes much higher that you start to feel unwell. This is one reason why it is never enough just to sail along on the same dose of insulin day by day without checking blood glucose levels or HbA1c levels. You may have a constantly raised blood glucose, which can be quietly doing you damage without you knowing anything about it.

In fact, if you have been 'hyper' for long periods you may not recognize how unwell you have been until your glucose levels are brought under stricter control. You then find out, perhaps for the first time in years, how it feels to be truly well. People with poorly controlled Type 1 diabetes are often hyperglycaemic all the time, with spikes of even higher blood glucose levels after meals.

Once the 'hyper' symptoms start, though, you do become very aware of them. An early one is blurred vision, as the lens in the eye changes shape. High glucose levels are a fertile breeding ground for bacteria, while at the same time they interfere with your defences against infection. So you are much more prone to infections wherever a body surface meets the environment – like the skin and lungs. Recurring boils that do not heal and repeated chest infections can be the first hint of both Type 1 and Type 2 diabetes.

Rising blood glucose levels interfere with the brain, dulling intellect and the ability to concentrate and making people lethargic and sleepy. The higher-than-normal blood glucose levels also overpower the kidney's ability to retain the glucose in the bloodstream, so it appears in the urine. The more glucose there is in the urine, the more water the kidneys have to excrete along with it, so hyperglycaemia brings with it excessive urine excretion. In short, you pass more urine more often than normal, day and night. The depletion of your body water makes you thirsty, so you drink more, too.

Urine is not a matter of water alone, however. It contains minerals such as sodium, potassium and magnesium that are essential to the workings of many organs, including the muscles. So as you pass more urine, you lose more minerals, too. Lacking essential minerals, the muscles become less efficient, so you develop cramp and weakness on top of the tiredness and lethargy.

If this process continues for any length of time, because your body no longer has access to glucose as its source of energy (it is all trapped in the circulation and can't get to the tissues), it uses its stored fatty tissue instead. This produces weight loss which can be quite drastic. In undiagnosed Type 1 it can be several stones (15 kg or more) in a month or two. By then your urine is full of ketones, as well as glucose.

Finally, if the diabetes is completely out of control, you become dehydrated; with glucose levels rising steeply, you become breathless and lose consciousness, lapsing into coma.

Hopefully, no person with diagnosed Type 1 diabetes should reach this state. Long before it is reached, the initial symptoms of blurred vision, lethargy, poor concentration, thirst and excessive urine production, cramps and weakness, and the smell of ketones in the breath should have made the diagnosis obvious, and the correct treatment should have been started. But it is as well for everyone with diabetes and their families to be very well acquainted with the possibility and to know exactly what to do when confronted with it.

Sometimes it is easy to miss. For example, it could be mistaken for drunkenness, especially after people have had a drink or two and forgotten to take their insulin. People with diabetes have also been known to forget to take their insulin with them on a journey, and decided to take the risk of missing a dose or two. Hyperglycaemia can creep up on them without them noticing, and they can quickly become too confused to tell people about it. Teenagers may deliberately do without their insulin dose as an act of rebellion against their disease and the discipline of managing it. They, too, can be mistakenly diagnosed as drunk at, say, a party, when the real cause is lack of insulin and consequent hyperglycaemia.

It is incumbent on everyone with diabetes and their families to be as expert as their doctors in recognizing the signs of early hyperglycaemia and correcting it as soon as possible. That means people with Type 1 diabetes should always make sure they have their insulin delivery kit – and preferably their blood glucose monitoring kit as well – with them at all times. They should also wear a Medicalert disc so that anyone finding them in a semi-conscious state knows who they are and whom to contact for help.

Ketoacidosis

Ketoacidosis (or ketosis) is the end-result of neglected hyperglycaemia. Every Type 1 diabetic must always be aware of how it feels to become ketotic, because recognizing it and reversing it in time can save their lives. As explained earlier, when the body is unable to use glucose as a source of energy it has to turn for energy directly to the fat stored in the fatty tissues. Even people who do not have diabetes but have not eaten for a day or so, and have therefore depleted their liver and muscle stores of glycogen (see page 11), must start breaking down their body's fat stores. It is the mechanism we use when we are starving.

As explained earlier, using fat directly in this way (we normally convert it into glucose first, then use insulin to pump it into the organs and tissues) leads to ketones as a waste product. Ketones build up in the bloodstream, and the excess appears in the urine, in which it can be detected by simple 'strip' tests. Normal urine, passed by people without diabetes who are not starving, or by people with diabetes under good control, does not contain any detectable ketones.

In poorly controlled or undiagnosed Type 1 diabetes (with too little insulin activity, too much carbohydrate intake, or both), rising blood ketone levels lead to trouble. This is because ketones are acid. The body's metabolism is organized so that it works most efficiently when all the body's fluids (in the blood and in the fluid in and around the tissues and organs, including the brain and muscles) are slightly alkaline (the opposite of acidic). As the ketone levels build up, the body's ability to keep the acid-alkaline balance precisely as it should be (for the technically minded, a pH level of around 7.3 to 7.4) fails, and the body becomes 'acidotic' (the pH drops, so that in extreme cases it can fall below 7.0).

33

In this state of ketoacidosis, none of the organs works well. The brain, liver and kidneys start to fail, so you become tired, sleepy, feel sick and may even vomit. Because your kidneys excrete far more fluid than normal, you quickly become parched. Your mouth dries up and you breathe very deeply (doctors call this 'Kussmaul' breathing). If this state of affairs continues, you will become unconscious. This is a diabetic coma.

Before we had insulin, ketoacidosis and coma were the usual cause of death in diabetes. It takes about 24 hours to progress from the start of ketoacidosis to coma, so there should always be time to prevent it from becoming a serious threat to life, as long as the early signs are recognized and they are properly treated.

How do you recognize if you are slipping into ketoacidosis? The initial change is becoming more thirsty and passing more urine than normal, particularly if your blood glucose level is over 17 mmol/L. If at any time you have a blood glucose level this high you must check your urine for ketones. If the result is positive, then check again in 3 to 4 hours. If ketones are still present you must contact your clinic urgently for advice, unless you have specific instructions designed just for you under these circumstances.

The numbers of cases of ketoacidosis are, thankfully, very low among people with Type 1 diabetes these days. This is partly because they are now under regular management. All people with diabetes in Britain should be under a general practice or hospital diabetes management team, and should therefore be well aware of the problem and how to avoid it. However, it won't do any harm to list the ways ketoacidosis can occur and how to avoid them.

Too Much Food or Too Little Exercise

The most common causes of ketoacidosis are still too much food or too little exercise. Problems arising from either can be prevented by keeping to regular eating and exercise patterns, and by increasing your insulin dose when you eat more or exercise less. By how much to change the insulin dose may be a matter of trial and error, with the guidance of your diabetes specialist nurse or doctor. Each person is different, and it would not be useful here to describe dose schedules in detail, as what suits one person may well not suit another.

Developing ketoacidosis may be a gradual process, as your insulin needs may change as time passes. One way of preventing its onset is to monitor your blood glucose levels carefully: if over days and weeks they are gradually rising, you may have to increase your insulin dose by between two and eight units per injection. This, too, should be discussed with your diabetes nurse or doctor.

Forgetting to Take an Insulin Dose
A single forgotten insulin dose isn't likely to produce ketoacidosis. In any case this can be put right according to simple rules. For example, if you are injecting insulin twice daily, and remember that you have forgotten your morning dose before mid-day, take between half and two-thirds of the dose immediately. If you don't remember it until the evening, then check your blood glucose and get on your usual diabetes 'hotline' to discuss the appropriate dose with a nurse or doctor. Most people nowadays take four injections a day: forgetting one of them should not cause any serious problem, and there is no need to adjust the next dose.

During Illness or Times of Stress
Probably the most difficult time for someone with Type 1 diabetes is during another illness, particularly an infection or when under physical or mental stress. This can also bring on ketoacidosis if not managed correctly. Being in an accident, undergoing an operation, having anxiety or depression, or even something as simple as a common cold or flu can push up your blood glucose levels. How much higher blood glucose gets varies widely from person to person, so again it isn't easy to give precise instructions here on how to raise the insulin dose to compensate.

Under these circumstances the rule is to check your blood glucose level once every four hours or so while you are ill or under unusual stress. You may have to increase your insulin levels by anywhere from four units to double your usual dose, depending on how high your blood glucose levels are. Experience will tell you how much extra you need, and as always be guided by your diabetes nurse or doctor.

A particular risk is posed by an illness that stops you eating, makes you vomit or gives you diarrhoea. Gastro-enteritis, for example, may give you all three. It is vital that you do *not* stop your insulin: just because you cannot take in food does not mean that you must lower your insulin dose accordingly. This is a mistake often made by people newly diagnosed with diabetes. Instead, you must measure your blood glucose level more often than usual, and increase your insulin accordingly if it is climbing. At the same time you should try to swallow fluids that contain carbohydrates.

Foods that are useful sources of fast glucose during illness include glucose itself, sugar, jams, marmalades and honey, undiluted fruit squashes and juices, lemonade, tinned milk puddings, drinking chocolate, and powders such as Complan and Build-up normally reserved for invalids.

If while you are ill, and particularly if you are being sick and are getting dehydrated, you find that your urine is positive for ketones, then you must immediately contact your usual diabetes expert (usually via a hotline). If this continues for more than four or five hours, then get someone to take you to the accident and emergency department of your local hospital.

If you are isolated and cannot get into hospital, and you know your diabetes is getting much worse, with ketones and a rising blood glucose, then until you can reach medical help follow the following rules:

- inject 4 units of a fast-acting insulin (such as Actrapid, Humulin-S, or lispro) once an hour
- check your blood glucose once an hour until it falls to normal for you
- drink at least a pint (600 ml) of water every hour until you return to normal

If you have the type of 'brittle' diabetes that means you have such problems fairly often, and live where it is difficult to reach professional help easily, it is a good idea to place the above list in a prominent place where everyone in the house can see it. They can all be taught how to give you your injections, too, so that they can help even when you are too confused or sleepy to do it yourself.

Hypoglycaemia

Hypoglycaemia is likely to happen when the blood glucose drops below 3 mmol/L (millimoles per litre – in North America this is measured as mg/dl or milligrams per decilitre; 3 mmol/L = 50 mg/dl). Hypoglycaemia produces hunger, dizziness, sweating, trembling, slurred speech, faintness, confusion and palpitations (a fluttering feeling in the chest due to fast heartbeats). If not treated urgently, the person loses consciousness and may even convulse (have a fit).

Everyone with Type 1 diabetes must be able to recognize how they feel when becoming hypoglycaemic. Your pattern of symptoms is unique to you, and you must be able to recognize them early so that you can reverse the hypoglycaemia before you are unable to do so. Your doctors may even have you undergo a 'hypo' deliberately while in the safety of the clinic, so that you can later recognize your symptoms and know how to deal with them efficiently.

One particular type of 'hypo' is the type that happens when you are asleep. If you have spent a restless night, perhaps having had a nightmare, and wake with a headache, you probably have had a hypo in the small hours. Paradoxically, you may find that your blood glucose the following morning is higher than usual. This is despite urine tests taken at the same time being free of glucose, but positive for ketones. To prevent such night-time hypos, you should have a bedtime snack.

Patterns of hypos may change over the years. In particular you may lose the first warning signs (usually sweating and trembling). You need to be alert to this change and to recognize the other signs. If you find your early warning signs are becoming less obvious, you may need to lower your insulin dose or change your insulin type. See later for more details about insulin use.

Delaying or Missing Meals
The main causes of hypoglycaemic attacks are delaying or missing meals after giving yourself an insulin dose. You should be very strict about regular mealtimes, and about your regular snacks between meals and before sleeping.

Accidental Overdose
Other causes include an accidental overdose of insulin. If you realize quickly that this has happened, you can usually prevent a serious hypo by taking extra glucose. If it is a high overdose (say twice your usual dosage or more), you must tell your doctor at once.

Unplanned Physical Activity
Unplanned extra physical activity can also induce hypo attacks, so everyone with Type 1 diabetes should carry a stock of glucose (such as Dextrosol tablets) or lump sugar in a pocket or handbag. Sometimes an action as simple as running for a bus or having to climb stairs when a lift is out of order may precipitate a hypo.

Alcohol
Finally, there is alcohol. Moderate to heavy drinking can interfere with

the body's control of the balance between blood glucose and insulin, so that it can increase the risk of a hypo even when you have otherwise eaten normally and taken the right dose of insulin. People with Type 1 diabetes should never binge-drink, and should always eat whenever they are drinking.

How to Avoid a Hypoglycaemic Attack

As repeated hypo attacks can harm the brain, they should be avoided as far as possible. The easiest way to do so is to carry on your person, all the time, a packet of glucose (dextrose) tablets. Even if the attack is a mild one, a tablet chewed at the first symptom can be essential to prevent it becoming more serious. A more severe attack can be quickly corrected by a drink of sweetened milk and a sweet biscuit. If you become too drowsy too quickly to deal with the problem yourself, the instructions on your Medicalert bracelet should be clear enough for people near you to feed you a sweet drink before you lose consciousness. You should make sure that your immediate friends and family all know how to recognize a 'hypo' and understand how to deal with it.

Hypostop is a glucose-rich jelly in a tube that can be squeezed like toothpaste into the mouth of people in hypo attacks, and if necessary rubbed on to the gums. In an emergency, if the hypo is causing the person to lapse into unconsciousness, then a doctor will inject glucose solution into a vein. People who are prone to repeated hypo episodes may be prescribed injections of glucagon, a hormone that has the opposite effect to insulin. It comes in the form of ampoules in a kit, with which friends and family must make themselves familiar. It is given as a 1-milligram injection of 1-millilitre solution into the thick muscle just below the shoulder on the outside of the upper arm. People coming round after a glucagon injection often feel sick, but the feeling clears over the next hour or so.

A point that cannot be made too strongly is that repeated hypo attacks should be avoided, because of the danger of long-term brain damage. In the past, when insulin injections were given only once or twice a day as a mixture of short-acting and long-acting preparations, people tended to tolerate the odd hypo as the price to pay for keeping their blood glucose levels as low as possible.

This is no longer the case. Today's treatment involves several injections of different types of insulin throughout the day, planned to fit with small and frequent meals. Individual insulin doses are now lower than they were, and in the cases of well-controlled Type 1 diabetes blood levels of both insulin and glucose do not fluctuate nearly as widely as was common only a few years ago.

With the much better control of both insulin and glucose levels, hypo attacks should be a thing of the past for most people with Type 1 diabetes. If you are having them, and have been unable to control them yourself, then you must discuss it as a matter of high priority with a diabetes specialist.

Chapter Five

Eating Right

It would be great if insulin could just be swallowed, like other medicines, say, for arthritis, but it can't. Being a protein, it would just be broken down by the digestive juices. So it must be injected. Future approaches include the possibility of giving it by nasal spray, as there is evidence that substances like insulin can be absorbed by the delicate membranes lining the nose. One difficulty with that approach is that insulin doses must be precise for good control, and the ability of the nasal membranes to absorb proteins varies hugely, as for example if a person has an allergy such as hay fever, or a cold. No one has yet found a way of consistently directing insulin through the extra mucus and thickening produced by either of these problems.

So, for the foreseeable future the main way of delivering insulin to people with Type 1 diabetes will be insulin injections. However, there are many forms of insulin, and different ways of getting them through the skin. Each diabetes specialist has his or her own favourites. This chapter describes them, hopefully without bias, so that you can compare your own method with others. More important, it gives practical hints on how to achieve the optimum control of your diabetes by combining your eating (I hate to use the word diet) and exercise habits with the most effective insulin doses and delivery systems.

Eating Wisely

To the general public, the word 'diet' has, over the years, acquired a slightly pejorative ring. It has been mainly linked to the need for cutting down calorie intake in people who are overweight. The obese 'go on diets' to lose weight, and it is clear to health care workers involved in obesity treatments that they are mostly unsuccessful. People switching to them may lose weight for a while, but the vast majority (the common figure quoted is 95 per cent) give them up and become just as obese as before within a year. So diets are seen as a temporary style of eating, usually restricting in some way, and often unpleasant or boring, used to achieve an aim and then cast aside as the aim is achieved.

For doctors and nurses, the word 'diet' in the context of diabetes has an entirely different meaning. It is a way of eating to which people with either Type 1 or Type 2 diabetes must adhere for the rest of their lives, and preferably very strictly. Not only is it a form of discipline, particularly for people with Type 1 diabetes, it must also be organized in relationship to insulin injections and to exercise habits. The three are interdependent, and must not be thought of as separate.

Do not let this bald statement of the facts dismay you. Sticking to strict rules about food does not mean that eating is less enjoyable. In fact, you may find that as you get used to the new habits food becomes much more enjoyable and tasty than before. One reason for this is that your new choices of food have more subtle tastes, not drowned out by the addition of sugar (nor, for that matter salt, about which more later).

I speak from my own experience. When I discovered my tendency towards Type 2 diabetes, I stopped adding sugar to my tea and coffee. As I had always had a sweet tooth (not uncommon in 'pre-diabetes people' like myself) I thought it would take time to lose it. Not at all. Within days I was enjoying the real tastes, not drowned in sugar or milk, of many different teas and coffees, and enjoying them thoroughly. It was no problem to abandon desserts and sweets, biscuits, cakes and scones because the substitutes, fresh fruits and vegetables, different types of breads and different ways of cooking potatoes, pasta and rice, were much tastier and just as filling.

The other big change was in my timing of meals. Although as a potential Type 2 diabetes sufferer I did not have to fit in my eating schedule with insulin injections, it would have been easy to do so. Instead of my old habit of a light breakfast, a slightly more substantial lunch and a 'proper' meal in the evening, I quickly grew used to eating three moderate meals equally spaced throughout the day, making the last one a single course, finishing with a piece of fresh fruit.

I quickly realized that I very much enjoyed the radical change in my eating habits. I never ate so much that I felt full, felt much less hungry during the daytime, and started to lose weight. Within two months I had lost my extra 2 stone and felt great. I was no longer lethargic, had a much better sense of taste, had plenty of energy and was eating much less, and enjoying what I ate. More than 20 years later I am still eating in the same way, and am lucky enough to have remained fit (so far).

In no way could what I eat be called a 'diet' in the lay sense of the word, because it is enjoyable and not, to my mind, restrictive, although in the medical sense I had put myself on a diet suitable to Type 1 diabetes.

Here are its principles in more detail.

Everyone Benefits

First of all, everyone, with diabetes or not, would benefit from eating in this way. So if you are the one with diabetes in your family, why not get your family and friends to enjoy this healthy eating plan with you? It is difficult to be the only one in a family to be eating in one way, while all the others are tucking into chips, cakes and desserts. There is no need to buy special 'diabetic' foods, which are generally more expensive, and not necessarily better for you. A generation ago, people with diabetes were restricted largely to salads and special breads and rolls that tasted like cardboard. Thank goodness we know better now.

Let's start on a positive note. If you like Italian, Greek and Spanish food, you'll like being on a 'diabetic diet' – because Mediterranean cooking is almost completely compatible with diabetes. But don't let it go to your head. It is important not to eat too much, whatever you are eating, because becoming overweight (obese) can put people with either type of diabetes at greater risk than others of heart attacks and strokes.

Eating Rule 1: Avoid Sugary Foods

The first principle of eating well as a person with diabetes is to avoid foods and ingredients that, soon after they are swallowed, cause the blood glucose levels to rise steeply, and need a big surge of insulin to deal with the rise. These foods are defined as having a high 'glycaemic index' (glyc = glucose, aemic = in the blood). Your diabetes care team member responsible for looking after what you are eating, probably the dietician or the nurse, will have a comprehensive list of foods with a high glycaemic index. Suffice it to say here that these are mainly foods containing glucose, sugar or honey.

Some of these foods, because they taste sweet, are obvious. Jam, marmalade, honey, sweets, chocolate, fruit squashes, tinned or preserved fruits, cakes, baked goods of any sort, all have a high glycaemic index. But be careful about any prepared food. Look at the label and check if sugar or glucose features high on the list of ingredients or 'nutritional information' section. You may be surprised to learn that baked beans, well known to be high in fibre (7.7 g of fibre per 207 g serving) are even higher in sugar (12.4 g per 207 g serving). That doesn't mean you shouldn't eat baked beans, but at least, when you are taking your whole day's food intake into account, remember the contribution that baked beans make to your carbohydrate intake, and be prepared to adjust your treatment accordingly.

Artificial sweeteners are very much in vogue. So-called 'diet' fruit drinks are sweetened with saccharin, aspartame and other chemicals to make them more palatable to people wishing to retain their sweet tooth while slimming, or controlling their diabetes. Many also use sweeteners in their tea and coffee. I don't think artificial sweeteners help either group. I don't have figures to prove my point, but my experience over many years suggests to me that people who keep up their taste for sweet foods by using artificial sweeteners always fall by the wayside, and revert to their old sugary habits.

My patients who have deliberately decided to cut out all sweet-tasting foods (except for fresh fruit) have done much better and controlled their weight and their diabetes much better. As proof of that, look into the shopping trolleys of other customers next time you are at the supermarket. I bet that the fat customers have several bottles of diet coke or something similar in their trolley – and the thin customers prefer the 'real thing' or confine their sweet purchases to fruit.

People with diabetes who decide to cut out sweet foods can take comfort that it isn't socially unacceptable these days not to finish a meal with a dessert. It isn't as difficult to organize as, say, a diet for people with coeliac disease due to gluten allergy, or people with peanut allergy, or vegans. I've found, too, that, when someone tries to push a sweet or a cake on me, if I explain that I 'have a little trouble with sugar' it is perfectly acceptable, and the pressure disappears.

Another plus point about eating healthily in Type 1 diabetes is that there is hardly ever any need to count calories. Once you have got used to your new eating habits, it is fairly easy to know how much, and what, to eat to fit with your usual insulin dose. It comes with experience and training, and soon is second nature, much like learning to ride a bicycle as a child.

Eating Rule 2: Space Meals Regularly Throughout the Day

The spacing of meals regularly throughout the day is the next main principle of healthy eating. Many people with no experience of diabetes in the family still stick to the old habits of hardly any breakfast and two main meals each day. One is at lunchtime and one in the early evening, nowadays seated around the television with a tray on the knee instead of around the table with the rest of the family. The pros and cons of this latest social change in eating habits are still heatedly debated, but what matters to people with Type 1 diabetes is not *where* they eat, but *what they eat, how much, and how often.*

It is important not to miss breakfast, and to have three meals a day. If you stick to two (or even just one) large meals a day, much of that intake will be sugars, and your blood glucose levels will rise so steeply that you will need large amounts of injected insulin to cope with them. It is far better for you to have three relatively small meals, with little refined sugar in them, at regularly spaced times throughout the day. Then you can co-ordinate the food more easily with your insulin injections, so that you can keep the doses you need relatively low.

A 'meal' can mean anything from soup and a sandwich to meat, potatoes and vegetables, with a small dessert if you wish – just because I no longer eat them doesn't mean this is the right decision for everyone. What matters is that the load of food you eat at the meal coincides with the amount and type of insulin you have injected a few minutes beforehand. For a more difficult to control diabetes, a snack between meals may be needed to keep the blood glucose level within the accepted limits. A snack last thing at night to avoid a hypo while asleep may also be needed.

It is fine for people with Type 1 diabetes to have the occasional treat – say a larger than usual meal while out, but if you do so, remember to increase your insulin dose just *before* the meal to avoid hyperglycaemia. Take the advice of your diabetes nurse or dietician about the size of the increase you'd need with this type of meal.

Eating Rule 3: Plenty of Starch

Although it's important to avoid sugars, it's just as important to eat plenty of starches, the other source of carbohydrate in food. The main sources of starch are potatoes, bread, pasta, rice and other cereals. It takes longer for starches than for sugars to be digested down to glucose in the gut, so that after a starchy meal the blood glucose rise is much slower than after a sugary one. This means that less insulin has to be given to bring the glucose into normal blood levels, so that the blood glucose curve after the meal is much closer to normal.

Even then, care should be taken in cooking. For example, boiled potatoes produce a much smaller and slower rise in blood glucose than baked potatoes. Wholemeal and multi-grain breads, like boiled potatoes, have a low glycaemic index (see page 43), but white bread has similar glucose-raising properties to baked potatoes. The same goes for white rice and some breakfast cereals, such as cornflakes. Choose instead oat-based cereals, such as porridge, and less refined cereals such as brown rice, All-Bran and muesli. When choosing your breakfast cereals, keep these in mind; if in doubt, talk their properties over with your dietician and nurse.

Eating Rule 4: Remember Roughage

Fibre has been going in and out of diet fashion for 30 years, ever since Dr Denis Burkett, working in East Africa, proposed that it protected against bowel disorders. The experts are still arguing about that theory, but there is no argument against the proposal that fibre is an essential ingredient of the daily food for people with Type 1 diabetes. High-fibre foods have three advantages for people with diabetes: they reduce the rise in blood glucose after meals, so that less insulin is needed and the blood glucose curve is flatter. They help to lower blood cholesterol levels – a very important action for the long-term health of all people with diabetes, be it Type 1 or Type 2. And they tend to be very filling, so that they help you eat less without leaving you hungry. They can in this way help people reduce weight, and they also help in producing normal daily bowel movements.

Fibre is the relatively indigestible material of plant stems and cell walls. We do not produce the enzymes to break them down in our gut (unlike herbivores such as rabbits), so that fibre is not nutritious in itself, but it helps to slow down digestion of carbohydrates. This is the main reason for its ability to keep rises in blood glucose levels after meals to a minimum. Researchers have adopted this property to produce medicines, such as acarbose, about which there is more detail in the chapters on treating Type 2 diabetes.

Foods rich in fibre include multi-grain breads, long-grain brown rice, wholegrain pasta, green and yellow vegetables (such as peas, beans, lentils, carrots, turnips, beetroot, cabbages, sprouts and lettuce) and unrefined wholegrain cereals.

Eating Rule 5: Don't Overdo the Fats

It is understandable that people are confused by the different messages on fatty foods. On the one hand we hear a lot about how damaging animal fats are to the heart and circulation. On the other we hear how beneficial vegetable oils (like sunflower and rape seed) and fish oils (cod liver, halibut and oily fish in general) are to the same organs. So should the person with Type 1 diabetes do without dairy products and consume margarine instead?

There are two aspects of fats in food to be considered. The first, and of more immediate importance to people with diabetes, is that all fats, from whatever source, are a high source of calories. For example, 1 gram of carbohydrate (such as starch or sugar) provides 4 calories of energy. 1 gram of protein (for example lean meat, poultry and fish) also provides 4 calories. But 1 gram of fat or oil (of animal, fish or vegetable origin) provides 9 calories. Alcohol is close to fat in energy provision, in that 1 gram of pure alcohol gives you 7 calories.

So if you are fond of chips and oily foods, be aware that they are high-energy providers, and that you must take that into account in your diabetes control. Fats and oils are broken down into fatty acids by your digestive juices, to be taken up by the liver, which re-organizes them into the complex fats the body needs (like cholesterol, about which much more later). Fats essential to the function of fat-rich organs (like the brain, the nerve cells of which are full of, and surrounded by, fat) are transported to them in the bloodstream. So a basic minimum of fat is essential in our food to keep organs like the brain (and the liver itself, another organ that needs fats to function properly) healthy.

The problems arise when we eat too much fat for our needs. The excess is either stored in fat cells or converted to glucose and used to provide energy, in which, of course, insulin is involved. Excessive consumption of animal fats promotes the deposit of fat, in the form of cholesterol, in the walls of arteries, like the coronary arteries supplying the heart, or the cerebral arteries supplying the brain. There it causes inflammation and becomes the eventual focal point for the clots and haemorrhages that initiate heart attacks and strokes.

The process of laying down fats in the blood vessel walls is accelerated in people with poorly controlled diabetes. They should therefore avoid over-consumption of animal fats, not just because they may become overweight and have trouble with their diabetes control, but also because they would be putting themselves at a higher than necessary risk of a heart attack or stroke.

Vegetable and fish oils are different. They are less likely to lead to fatty deposits in the arteries, and there is good evidence that regularly eating foods rich in them actually protects you against heart attacks and strokes, because they promote the release of cholesterol deposits from the arteries.

So it should be good for you to eat oily fish (like mackerel, herring, tuna, sardines, pilchards, trout and salmon) around three times a week. And to grill them, rather than fry. When cooking, if you must enjoy a fry-up from time to time, use vegetable oils, but throw them away after they have been used twice. Preferably, use fresh oil each time. This is because repeated heating of vegetable oils changes their composition so that they behave in your body more like animal fats.

Eating Rule 6: Keep Slim

Your enthusiasm for oily fish and vegetable oils should not blind you to one of the most important messages for anyone with diabetes, Type 1 or Type 2. That is – do not allow yourself to become overweight. If you are already overweight, you must lose the excess pounds. For people without diabetes, being overweight is mostly just a nuisance. It is a cosmetic worry, perhaps, but as very many people in our society today are overweight, most people accept it and treat it as a minor problem that some day they may do something about.

For someone with diabetes, this attitude would be a big mistake. Being overweight raises insulin needs and makes it much more difficult to control your blood glucose levels. It is also linked to higher-than-normal blood levels of the fats (LDL-cholesterol and triglycerides, about which more later) which raise your risks of a heart attack or stroke. Obesity is linked, too, to high blood pressure, control of which is just as important as control of blood glucose (more about this later, too).

So, now that you have diabetes you must take control of your own weight, and the only way to do that is to organize not just your eating habits and insulin injections, but your exercise, too. If you are having trouble with your weight, discuss your eating and exercise habits in detail with your dietician and diabetes nurse. They will together draw up a programme that combines the right way to eat and to exercise so that you will lose the extra pounds. Don't be tempted to follow those crazy low-calorie diets repeated again and again in magazines. They are not for people with diabetes (I would claim they are not for any normal person), and they could badly interfere with your diabetes control. Trust your medical and nursing team and stick by their instructions.

As for exercise, it isn't necessary to go running or to join a gym, although if you enjoy them, by all means do so. Simple walking is often good enough to lose weight. A half-hour's brisk walk or swimming in the local pool, or an hour on a bicycle, every day will take a stone (7 kg) off in a year, as long as you don't eat more. In fact, regular exercise often curbs the appetite, helping you to eat less. After just a week or so, you will begin to feel much better and fitter.

How do you know if you are overweight? That's simple. Just look in a long mirror. You can surely judge for yourself whether you have a spreading middle or hips. There is a formula, however, by which you can judge whether you are veering towards the obese. It is the body mass index, or BMI.

For the BMI you must know your weight in kilograms and your height in metres and centimetres. Divide your weight by the square of your height, and you should get a figure between 20 and 25, the normal range for BMI. Under 20 and you are a little too thin. Over 25 you are a little overweight. Over 30 you are fat enough to be diagnosed as clinically obese. Take my example. I'm 12 stone 7 (78 kg) and 5 foot 10 (1.78 metres). 1.78 squared is 3.17, so my BMI is 78 divided by 3.17, which is 24.6. That is just under the upper limit for normal, so I'm not overweight, but I still feel that it is slightly too heavy for me, so I'll take a little more exercise and eat a little less until I have lost two to three more kilograms. The BMI chart shown here will show you precisely you relate to the norm, and how much weight you need to lose (or gain, if you are underweight) to get into the normal range.

Eating Rule 7: Alcohol

This is where you must discipline yourself especially strictly. Over the last few years the messages about alcohol have been confusing. In the early 1990s the idea of 'safe' amounts of alcohol was promoted, so that it became acceptable for men to drink 21 units and women to drink 14 units a week without doing themselves any long-term harm. It came to be that drinking up to that amount of alcohol was actually good for you – not the intended message at all.

Then the red wine message hit the lay press. It came from a study by Professor Jean-Marc Orgogozo and his team at Bordeaux University. I have met Professor Orgogozo, and like him a lot. He is a good scientist, and is not funded by any special interest groups, such as the winemakers.

He started his research with the idea that regular drinking of red wine from a very early age, as happens in his region, might be harmful, so he

Body Mass Index Chart

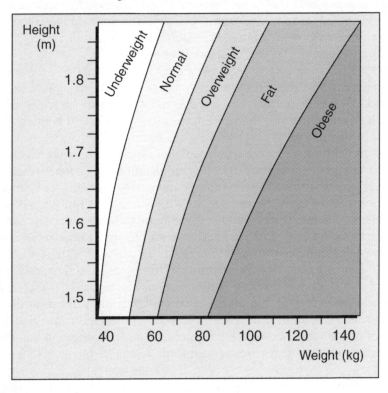

followed drinkers and non-drinkers for many years, noting what they died from and at what age. He was astonished to find that the wine drinkers outlived the non-drinkers by several years, and the difference persisted when he removed all the other possible influences that might have prolonged their lives (or shortened the non-drinkers' lives).

Clearly something in the red wine helped to protect drinkers from heart attacks and strokes. Was it the alcohol or a particular property of the wine, unrelated to its alcohol content? The academic argument continues: well-respected researchers in Edinburgh and in Munich have reported a similar 'saving of lives' by moderate drinking of whisky or beer. The figures are confirmed by surveys of millions of deaths reported to life assurance companies, in which it is certain that lifelong teetotallers tend to die a year or two *before* moderate drinkers.

So is a little alcohol each day a good thing for people with diabetes? Much depends on what you define as a little, and whether you can keep it to a little. The standard advice is to drink no more than two to three units of alcohol a day if you are a woman, and three to four if you are a man. A unit means a single measure of spirits (a 'half' in Scotland), a standard glass of wine, a small glass of fortified wine like sherry or port, or a half pint (250 ml) of beer – even less than that if it is a strong beer.

However, this advice is for the general population, not people with Type 1 diabetes. For you, the advice must be much more precise. To start with, alcohol is a high source of calories (remember, 1 gram gives you 7 calories), so you must take that into account when you are giving yourself your insulin. Secondly, too much alcohol drunk over even a moderate period can start to harm your liver, brain and peripheral nerves – the nerves that detect sensations (pain, touch, heat, cold, vibration, position sense) and initiate muscle action between your limbs and the spinal cord. If you regularly overdo your alcohol intake you are inviting liver, brain and nerve disease, and once they have been established, they are hard to reverse.

If you already have signs of peripheral neuropathy (your specialist will, hopefully, already have done the necessary tests described on page 26), even moderate amounts of alcohol can make it worse. A relatively minor loss of sensation in the fingers and toes can develop into constant pins and needles, numbness and an inability to tell when water is scalding hot or freezing cold. And, as peripheral nerves run to and from the genital area, one sign of diabetic neuropathy is impotence. Alcohol ruins the performance even of people without diabetes (read the gatekeeper scene in *Macbeth*): if you are a man with Type 1 diabetes, the combination of alcohol and neuropathy can leave you impotent long after the hangover has gone.

So it is wise for all people with Type 1 diabetes to keep their alcohol intake down to a minimum, say one or two units a day at most, and have several days a week alcohol-free. If you already have neuropathy, seriously consider if you can do without alcohol altogether.

However much you drink, make sure that you never do it on an empty stomach. Alcohol on an empty stomach can drive your blood glucose level down into the hypo region. If you must have a pre-meal drink, then have a starch-rich snack with it, such as a sandwich. That's important, too, at bedtime, if you like a small 'nightcap'. Don't have the drink on its own – have a savoury biscuit or a small sandwich with it. Otherwise you may have a hypo during the night, with its accompanying nightmares, restlessness and headache in the morning.

Chapter Six

Organizing Your Insulin

Insulin injections are classified by how fast they begin to act, and for how long they continue to act, after the injection. So they can be 'very fast-acting', 'short-acting', 'intermediate-acting' or 'long-acting'. They are also classified according to their origins. Until recently insulins have been prepared from extracts of animal pancreas, so that the earlier insulins taken from cows were 'beef' insulins and the later ones almost always came from pigs (porcine insulins).

Each animal species produces its own specific insulin, slightly different chemically from all the others. Porcine insulin is chemically closer to human insulin than beef insulin, and is thought to cause fewer allergic reactions. Human insulin is either porcine insulin chemically modified to mimic the chemistry of human insulin or a synthetic insulin made by the latest in DNA technology, details of which are outside the scope of this book. One form of human insulin, for example, is made from an insulin 'precursor' chemical found in yeast cells.

Just because it is the same substance as is produced by human beings does not mean that human insulin is necessarily better at controlling your blood glucose than porcine insulin. When it was first made available, many people who were switched to it from porcine insulin found that they didn't get on with it so well. Some found, for example, that they lost the warning signs of hypo attacks. That led to sudden loss of consciousness in some people who had not had hypos for years.

That period is thankfully behind us. Staff in diabetes clinics and general practice are well aware of the advantages and pitfalls of the different forms of insulin, and are able to give personal advice to every Type 1 diabetic that is tailored to them and their particular insulin needs. So you may be given porcine or human insulin: what matters is not the type you are prescribed, but whether it does the job with the fewest side-effects for you. And the job is to maintain your blood glucose level as close to normal as possible.

Very rapidly-acting insulin (lispro) starts to work on blood glucose levels within 5 to 15 minutes of the injection, so that it is given immediately before, during or immediately after a meal. Its main effect takes place at around two hours after the injection, and although there is still some glucose-lowering activity for up to six hours, its action is shorter than that of soluble insulins.

Short-acting insulins are the soluble (acid or neutral) insulin preparations. They look clear in the syringe. They begin to act between 20 and 30 minutes after injection, the peak effect being at around 3 hours later, the activity lasting for 6 to 8 hours depending on the dose. You would have to take three doses evenly spaced out throughout a 24-hour period if you wanted to use short-acting insulins on their own to control your blood glucose properly.

Longer-acting insulins are one answer to this inconvenience. The action of insulin can be lengthened to between 12 and 36 hours by combining it with various proteins. Examples include isophane insulin and insulin zinc suspension. They look cloudy in the syringe, and need only to be given once or twice a day, provided that they control blood glucose levels well by doing so.

In people without diabetes, insulin levels in the blood fluctuate widely in response to meals. This can't be mimicked by either more frequent injections of shorter-acting insulins or by less frequent injections of longer-acting insulins on their own. What is needed is a mixture of the two – the shorter ones for mealtimes, when you need the 'spike' of insulin, and the longer ones for in between meals when you want to keep the blood glucose on a level keel with a steady supply of insulin.

To answer this need, manufacturers have provided 'biphasic' insulins, mixtures of insulins with different lengths of action to fit in with your own pattern of blood glucose. They contain different proportions of shorter- and longer-acting insulins, so that you can adjust the speed of onset and the length of action of the insulin combination to suit you. You should find your brand(s) of insulin in the table below.

Your diabetes medical and nursing team will work out with you what should be best for your particular eating and lifestyle habits and your weight. They will then monitor your progress closely, with regular blood glucose and HbA1c measurements, and fine-tune the dosage for a few weeks. When they think the control is as good as they and you, working together, can achieve, you can then settle into a normal routine of insulin injections with an appropriate eating and exercise plan.

Practical Points About Insulin Injections

The timing of insulin injections is crucial. With the exception of lispro

insulin (Humalog) which as mentioned above should be given immediately before, during or after a meal insulin should be given 15 to 30
minutes before meals. Lispro is helpful if the meal is unexpected or you
do not know how much food there will be.

Table of Insulins

Fastest action:	Action starts within minutes	Lispro Aspart
Soluble insulins:	Action starts after 30 minutes (peaks from 2 to 4 hours lasts up to 8 hours)	Neutral Actrapid Velosulin Humulin S Insuman Rapid
Intermediate acting:	Action starts after 1 hour (peaks from 4 to 12 hours lasts 16 to 35 hours)	Isophane Insulin zinc suspension
Proprietary names include:		Lente Lentard Monotard Ultratard Humulin Zn Humulin I Insulatard Insuman Basal
Longest acting:	Protamine zinc insulin (now rarely used as it cannot be given in the same syringe as other insulins).	

Giving an insulin injection too long before eating may give you a
hypo, as the insulin acts *before* the new glucose from the food enters
the bloodstream. This is particularly important if some of the injection
is short-acting. Giving insulin (apart from lispro) too near the mealtime
may allow the glucose from the food to rise too high in the bloodstream
before the insulin starts to work. So the timing should be just right.

Although it would be good to be able to return to the old days of a
once-daily injection of a biphasic insulin (see above), it would not give
good enough control. So most people have to give themselves several
injections a day. Some people with Type 2 diabetes (see Chapter Eleven) may need a longer-acting insulin injection last thing at night so

that their early morning blood glucose is near-normal.

Twice-daily biphasic insulin, given before breakfast and before the evening meal, may work well. Most people on twice-daily insulin need a higher dose in the morning than in the evening, and must eat small snacks between meals and at night. There is a growing tendency today, however, for people to give themselves short-acting insulin doses before each meal – normally three times a day – and combining that with a medium- or long-acting dose at bedtime. A few people will add a small dose of medium-acting insulin mid-morning. This gives them the chance to change doses to cope with different meal sizes and exercise levels, and to be much more flexible from day to day in their mealtimes. It also lets them do without the between-meals snacks, though they should always take that last-thing-at-night snack to avoid night-time hypos.

It takes time to master all the details of which kind of insulin you should have, at what dose, and how often, and how to adjust all of these with changing mealtimes and exercise sessions, but it is worth it. Once you have done so, you will find that the better quality of life this mastery gives is worth the bother of the extra injections each day.

Giving the Injections

All syringes are now of the disposable plastic type, and most have the needles fixed to them. They are designed to be thrown away after single a use, but they can be used several times if they are looked after properly. Do not do this, however, before talking about it with your doctor or diabetes nurse, who will give you specific advice on how to keep it scrupulously clean. The key is to place it back in its plastic cover without rinsing it in any way, and storing it in the refrigerator until it is needed again. In any case, throw it away after it has been used five times, or before that if the needle is blunt.

Syringes come in 30-, 50- and 100-unit sizes and may differ in their markings, so become expert in recognizing your dose. If the type or size of the syringe is changed, get very clear instructions from your diabetes nurse on the dose you need and how this looks on the syringe scale.

To draw the right amount of insulin into the syringe, first pull back the 'plunger' of the syringe so that it takes in air to the mark of the dose of insulin you are giving yourself. Then insert the needle through the top of the insulin bottle and inject the air into it. With the syringe pointing up vertically, the bottle upside down, and the tip of the needle below the liquid surface, withdraw the plunger slowly and the insulin should appear in the syringe without bubbles in it. If you do get bubbles, push the plunger in again until the bubbles escape, then withdraw it again, so that it is bubble-free. Then take the needle from the bottle. If you are taking both a short-acting and a long-acting insulin, draw in the clear (short-acting) insulin first, then the cloudy (long-acting), into the same syringe, and inject it immediately.

Many people now use insulin pens. In Scandinavia, for example, more than 85 per cent of all insulin-using people with diabetes of either type use pens, rather than syringes. Pens either come with a cartridge of 150 or 300 units of insulin that you load into them, or are preloaded with insulin by the manufacturer. Preloaded pens are disposed of after the insulin is used up. In either form of pen, you 'dial up' your dose before the injection. The needles can be changed as they become blunt. If you use a pen, make sure you have a spare, in case you break or lose the original. It happens!

Whatever you use, pen or syringe, how and where to give the injection is important. We used to advise cleaning the skin first with spirit, using cotton wool or a swab. Now we know that this is unnecessary. It is not only inefficient at sterilizing the skin (which was why people used to do it), but frequent swabbing of the skin with spirit or alcohol toughens it so that it is harder to slip a needle through it, and it makes needles blunt faster.

The insulin should be deposited under the skin, not into it, but not so deep that it gets into the underlying muscle. So you should use needles that are the right length for you. The standard needles are 12 millimetres (half an inch) long, but you may find shorter needles (8 mm or 3/8 in, 5 mm or 1/4 in) more appropriate. Whatever the length of the needle, you should pinch up a piece of skin into a fold, then push the whole length of the needle into it, holding it at right angles to the body surface. Then press the plunger straight down in one movement, making sure that all the dose is delivered before quickly withdrawing the needle.

Use different sites for your injections in rotation, never repeating the injection in exactly the same spot. If you must use the same area of skin in succession, at least make the next injection site more than an inch (2.5 cm) away from the previous one. Repeating an injection at the same spot can cause overgrowth of the tissues at that spot, a condition called *lipohypertrophy*. This may be to do with the fact, recently discovered, that insulin may stimulate growth of tissues if repeatedly injected into the same spot.

In a Finnish study reported in December 2000 of 100 people with Type 1 diabetes, 65 per cent of them had injection site complications, most of them lipohypertrophy of the tissues under the abdominal skin. Most of these people continually used a very small area for their injections (not much bigger than a postage stamp, according to the investigating doctors), and most had relatively poor glucose control (HbA1c more than 8.5 per cent). Unbelievably, many of the Finns had injected through a buttonhole into their abdominal skin because it was considered convenient. They were getting repeated injections in exactly the same place.

Less often than hypertrophy, repeated injections in the same place may lead to a hollowing out of the skin and tissues underneath. This process, called *atrophy*, is due to shrinkage of the fatty tissues under the skin due to their constant exposure to high concentrations of insulin. It is thought to be less common than in the past because insulins are now purer than they used to be.

You will have your own preferred injection sites – they vary from the outer upper arm to the front of the thighs and the skin of the lower abdomen. Some people find that the insulin takes effect sooner if they use the upper arm rather than the leg; others find the abdominal skin more efficient. It is difficult to see why this should be: you will find out the areas that suit you best as you vary the sites yourself.

Injections, despite what some diabetes specialists may say, are not painless. They sting a bit. But if you have a burning sensation or pain after an injection, or the site becomes red afterwards, you should tell your doctor or diabetes nurse. You may not be injecting yourself correctly, or may be developing an allergy to the insulin preparation you are using.

One final point which may seem obvious but is important. When visiting the pharmacist for your new prescription of insulin or syringe or pen, take your old ones with you, so that you are sure that the repeat prescription is exactly the same as the last one. Check the trade name of the insulin, and its colour code and strength, and check that the pen or syringe has the same dose markings on it. This will help to avoid errors in dosage, in type of insulin, and in delivery. It can be so easy to be lulled into a routine, and fail to notice a subtle difference in packaging that is potentially dangerous.

Chapter Seven

Tests and Targets

Not so long ago, the only testing people with Type 1 diabetes did for themselves was for glucose in the urine. It involved sticking strips of paper into urine samples and watching for the colour change. The results were given in terms of plusses – 0 if there was no glucose, + for a minor amount, ++ for a moderate amount, and +++ for severe glycosuria (glycosuria is simply a medical term for glucose in the urine). People and their doctors were expected to judge how well-controlled the diabetes was from diaries containing daily test results.

This type of testing has been consigned to the past, and rightly so, because the amount of glucose in the urine is at best a very rough guide to what is going on in the blood. Today we recognize that the only way to control diabetes correctly is to use blood glucose tests. That's why you are issued with blood glucose-testing gear and are asked to fill in the results accurately day by day. It is a shame that you must add daily finger pricks to your insulin injections – people with diabetes must put up with a lot of episodes of discomfort to look after themselves – but it is very definitely worth it in the long run.

Blood Glucose Testing

The first object of all blood glucose testing is to obtain a fresh drop of blood easily, without coaxing by pressure, from some skin site. Many manuals suggest the fleshy skin of the fingertips should be used. This can be very painful, and it is important to rotate the fingertips used to prevent a frequently used finger from becoming painful and even scarred. My own preference is the back of a finger, between the base of the nail and the knuckle. It is less sensitive to pain and bleeds just as profusely as the fingertip. An ear lobe is another good substitute.

It is important to get plenty of blood welling up from the 'jab' with the lancet, as the strip used for testing must be thoroughly covered with the blood. If you have to squeeze the finger to get the blood out, you may not get an accurate result.

Whatever strip test is used, you must time exactly the moment the blood touches the strip. If you are using a meter (most people use meters today), the timer button must be pressed at exactly the right time. If you are instructed to wipe the strip free of blood, then you must time that accurately, too. Some meters do this automatically.

If you are in any doubt about how to use your meter or how to check that your blood glucose testing is accurate, go through it in detail with your diabetes nurse or doctor. Remember that if you get a 'funny' reading, it may be the meter that is wrong, not your blood glucose. If you suspect that you are getting incorrect readings, use the check fluids provided with the machine as a comparison. It is a good idea, too, to have your machine tested regularly against standard blood samples in the laboratory.

When to Test

All people with Type 1 diabetes should measure their blood glucose levels at least once a day, and note them down in a daily diary for review by their diabetes nurses or doctors. This is the only way to know whether you are keeping your glucose levels as close as possible to the normal pattern. The tests should be done at different times each day, so that an overall picture can be presented. In effect, you are creating a blood glucose 'curve' whose points are collected over a month or so.

Why is this so important? The lower you keep your glucose levels, the better your chance of avoiding the major complications of diabetes – heart attack, stroke, kidney failure, blindness, diabetic gangrene, repeated infections and peripheral neuropathy.

Your Target Blood Glucose Levels

People who do not have diabetes have a fasting blood glucose level (taken first thing in the morning, around 12 hours after their last meal or snack) of around 5 millimoles per litre (mmol/L) or, in American usage, 90 milligrams per decilitre mg/dl. After eating a meal, their normal insulin response prevents their blood glucose from rising above 8 mmol/L (145 mg/dl).

In untreated or poorly controlled diabetes, blood glucose levels can rise well above 20 mmol/L (360 mg/dl) after a meal. The aim of most diabetes clinics is to get their patients' blood glucose levels down to between 4 and 7 mmol/L (70-125 mg/dl) before meals and between 7 and 10mmol/L (125-180 mg/dl) between one and two hours after meals. With figures like these, their HbA1c will almost certainly be below 7.5 per cent, a figure linked with a relatively low risk of later strokes, heart attacks and kidney failure.

Although they are not quite as low as the figures in people who do not have diabetes, they are fairly strict targets for people with diabetes who do not start to feel unwell with 'hyper' symptoms (see page 31) until their blood glucose levels are persistently above 14 mmol/L (250 mg/dl).

These strict targets are there for good reason: it is essential for all people with diabetes, of either main type, to understand that they cannot judge how well their diabetes is controlled by how they feel. You may feel well, but in fact be badly controlled and be open to severe health risks.

How to Achieve Good Control

Having Type 1 diabetes is different from having any other illness, because you become the manager of your own treatment. If you have read everything this far, you will have accepted that you must do everything you can to keep your blood glucose under control, 365 days and nights a year, and 366 in leap years. You, and only you, can do that. Your doctors and nurses can advise, but only you can put the treatment into practice.

Your main problem is that your life may vary from day to day, and with it your insulin requirements. If you had a normal pancreas, it would do all the work for you, altering your insulin output perfectly according to the food you have eaten. But you don't have a normal pancreas: you have to do all its work for it.

So to repeat the eating advice given a few pages ago, you must have three regular (if small) meals every day, and if necessary snacks between them and at bedtime. There is no harm in going out for a meal, as long as you plan beforehand. Take your blood glucose testing kit with you, and test after it. You will then know whether you have altered your pre-meal dose correctly, and whether you have to give yourself an extra dose of fast-acting insulin to counter a very high blood glucose level. It will also allow you to change your insulin injection accordingly the next time.

You should plan ahead like this for all conditions in which blood glucose is likely to rise abnormally, such as during times of physical and emotional stress and infections. Don't wait for the glucose to go up steeply – foresee the difficulty and increase the dose of insulin accordingly.

61

After that, measure your blood glucose and see if you adjusted the dose closely enough.

Exercise poses the opposite problem. If you are planning strenuous exercise (like tennis, squash, fast walking, running or, as in Sir Steven Redgrave's case, Olympic rowing) decrease your insulin dose. The change may be as little as four units, or as much as half your usual dose: only you can know, from your own experience of doing so and checking your blood glucose levels afterwards. You may also need to take extra glucose beforehand and during the exercise, to make sure you don't develop a 'hypo'. Taking extra glucose and less insulin are not alternatives but complementary measures.

It is important, too, to understand which dose of insulin affects which blood glucose test. For example, if you are giving yourself two doses of insulin each day, the morning dose affects the blood glucose level not only at midday, but also just before the evening meal. If the evening pre-meal blood glucose level is too high (persistently above 7 mmol/L), you may have to consider three insulin doses a day or a higher morning dose of longer-acting insulin. Similarly, the evening insulin dose affects the pre-breakfast blood glucose level the next morning. If that is too high, then you may need a larger evening dose of longer-acting insulin, or may need to switch to a different regimen, with perhaps more frequent doses of different insulins. If you are not achieving pre-meal blood glucose levels at or below 7 mmol/L, and after-meal levels at or under 10 mmol/L, you should discuss the possibility of better control with your diabetes team.

To Summarize

Please do undertake one or two blood glucose tests a day, and make note of them and the timing and amounts of your insulin injections, what you have eaten and the exercise you have done. If your control is not as it should be, your doctor and nurse should be able, from these data, to help you organize your insulin injections and your eating habits and exercise so that the control will improve. They won't mind you doing so, and they won't think you are wasting their time. Anything that can be done to improve your glucose control will put off the day that you develop more serious illness – and that will be a great saving in their time in the long run.

A final thought for this chapter – nowhere in this book have we yet mentioned smoking. People with either type of diabetes are mad to consider smoking even one cigarette a day. Why this is so is explained in Chapter Twelve. For the moment, however, it is enough to state that smoking can foul up not just the lungs but also the lives of everyone, but especially those with diabetes. So please don't smoke, ever. Just following this simple piece of advice could save your life.

Part Three
Living with Type 2 Diabetes

Chapter Eight

A Global Problem

In the early 1900s the Pima Indians living in the semi-desert lands of the southwestern United States were a healthy people. They were poor and only just managed to scrape a living, but photographs taken at the time show them to have been slim and fit.

By the 1960s they were a very different people. With the coming of industry and the loss of their traditional lifestyles, the grandchildren of those early 20th-century Native Americans grew up to be obese men and women, half of whom have Type 2 diabetes. Instead of the so-called civilized world bringing them better health and longer life, they are dying much earlier than their grandparents from strokes, kidney failure and heart attacks. These were illnesses that were, along with their diabetes, virtually unknown to their grandparents. The Pima who have remained physically active, stuck to their old ways and/or stayed slim have not developed diabetes, and do not die early.

The Pima are not alone. While they were developing their Type 2 diabetes, exactly the same was happening on the other side of the world to the Nauraun islanders of the South Pacific. 1 Today's Naurauns are much fatter than their ancestors, and have paid a very heavy price in that half now have Type 2 diabetes and the heart attacks and strokes that go with it.

The tragedies of the Pimas and the Naurauns are well known to medical students and doctors interested in diabetes all over the world, and have led to a much greater understanding of the processes that lead to Type 2 diabetes. The lessons learned from studying them have become a model for its treatment. They show that the main danger in Type 2 diabetes is not the disease itself, but its complications. As with Type 1 diabetes, it is easy to get by with reasonable control of the blood glucose, but the real skill is to keep the patient well into old age. This is what the rest of this book is about.

Why should Type 2 diabetes be so common in Native Americans and the Naurauns? The clue may lie in the fact that only two generations ago, they both survived by hunting and gathering food. They had to store fat in their tissues in times of plenty (mainly around the waist in men and around the hips in women); this enabled them to live on the fat and survive when food was scarce. In 1962, Dr J V Neel, writing in the American *Journal of Human Genetics*, suggested that there was an advantage to hunter-gatherers if their insulin activity directed more glucose to fat storage, and less to muscles, when they had plenty to eat. Their muscles would only take up substantial amounts of glucose when they needed it – for example actually during the hunt, when they were expending a lot of energy running.

In 1998, Dr G M Reaven took this theory further. He proposed that muscle proteins (the chemicals that make muscles contract and relax) are conserved better when there is less glucose around the muscle fibres. Hunter-gatherers, who need more than the usual amounts of insulin to drive glucose into their muscles and whose muscles take up glucose from the bloodstream only when they are exercising hard, may have healthier and stronger muscles than those with normal insulin-glucose responses.

So this 'insulin resistance', in which you need a much higher-than-usual insulin level in the blood to drive glucose levels into the muscles and therefore to bring down blood glucose levels, is an advantage for the hunter-gatherer. But it becomes a big disadvantage when the hunter-gatherer gives up his active lifestyle, becomes a near couch potato, and starts eating more. His genetics remain the same, so he creates more and more fat stores, his blood glucose remains high (because without exercise it takes a lot more insulin than in the rest of the population to bring it down) and he becomes obese. At the same time, his blood pressure rises, the excess fats in his bloodstream start to damage his circulation, and he becomes much more prone to heart attacks and strokes.

In the last few paragraphs I have used the male pronoun, because hunters were usually male. But the gatherers were women, and their lifestyles as the partners of the hunters were at least as strenuous physically, and often more so. For them, too, insulin resistance offered advantages in times of food scarcity and high physical activity. So female Pima Indians and Nauraun Islanders inherited the same pattern of insulin resistance as their male counterparts. Now that they also have more sedentary lives and have an abundance of food to eat, half of them, too, have Type 2 diabetes.

This background is quite different from the process that causes Type 1 diabetes. In people with a tendency to develop Type 1 diabetes, their pancreas has started off normally producing insulin, and rising glucose levels in the blood respond normally to it. As long as the pancreas continues to produce insulin, the relationship between insulin and glucose remains normal, so that the glucose in the blood is transferred in the usual way into the muscles, brain and all other tissues and organs.

Their Type 1 diabetes starts when some process causes insulin production to fail. We are still not sure what this process is. It seems to be an 'auto-immune' change, in which the body's immune system begins to mistake a protein produced normally by the body for a 'foreign' protein (as if it were the protein of an invading organism like a virus or bacterium, or an abnormal protein from a cancer cell). Once that occurs, the immune system destroys the protein (in this case insulin) as well as the cell system that makes it (the 'beta' cells of the pancreas).

So in Type 1 diabetes, the problem lies in the inability of the pancreas to produce the insulin that you need, because the cells that normally produce insulin have been destroyed by your body's own immune system.

There is no such problem in Type 2 diabetes. To begin with, the pancreas produces plenty of insulin. In fact it may over-produce it, so that blood levels of insulin are higher than normal. But even with this excess of insulin production, blood glucose levels remain slightly higher than normal, because the insulin 'pump' cannot drive the glucose from the blood into the tissues, where it should be used for energy, or back into the liver, where it should be stored as glycogen.

So the person with Type 2 diabetes, to start with, usually has relatively high blood glucose levels and high insulin levels, too. The beta-cells of the pancreas work overtime to produce more and more insulin to try to drive the glucose levels down, but eventually they give up the struggle, and the production of insulin falls. That is when the diabetes starts in earnest. The blood glucose levels become so high that they reach the levels seen in Type 1 diabetes, and much less insulin is produced in response to a glucose-containing meal.

However, the underlying biochemical differences between Type 1 and Type 2 diabetes may not be so clear-cut as the above explanation suggests. It used to be thought that there were distinct age differences between people with Type 1 and Type 2 diabetes. Type 1 diabetes was thought to start almost exclusively in childhood or the teenage years, and Type 2 diabetes in middle age and beyond. In fact, Type 1 is still often called 'juvenile' and Type 2 'maturity onset' diabetes. This is reflected in the other names for the two diseases – Type 1 as insulin-dependent and Type 2 as non-insulin-dependent.

These two classifications are less used in expert circles now, because teenage cases of Type 2 diabetes are becoming more common, and because many people with Type 2 diabetes need insulin to give them the optimum control of their blood glucose levels. And in 1993, Dr T Tuomi, Professor Paul Zimmet and their colleagues reported finding auto-immune antibodies against the production of insulin in between 10 and 15 per cent of older people labelled as having Type 2 diabetes. They were considered to have an 'incomplete Type 1 auto-antibody process' and an illness with the symptoms and properties of Type 2 disease.

Whatever the technical aspects underlying the disease, people may possess the elements of Type 2 diabetes for years before the imbalance between insulin and glucose levels (medically it is called insulin resistance) becomes bad enough to give obvious symptoms. The start of Type 1 diabetes in childhood is a rapid change in previously healthy children or teenagers. They become severely ill in a matter of days, with rapid weight loss, severe thirst and a great increase in the volume of urine, night and day. There is usually little doubt about the diagnosis within days of its onset.

In stark contrast, the onset of Type 2 diabetes is almost always very gradual. Typical Type 2 patients have put on, rather than lost, weight. They have taken little exercise: they probably have not done enough regular exercise to make them healthily breathless for some years. But when they have had to run for a bus or climb some stairs, they do get a bit 'short of breath'. They usually put that down to their age and excess weight, but do little about it.

It is only when they notice that they are sleepier than they used to be, say, in the middle of the day, especially after meals, and that they have started to get up at night to pass urine, and that they may be drinking a bit more than before, or that they are not seeing as well as they used to, that they ask to see their doctors.

They may not even do that. Many people with Type 2 diabetes are found because they have other, apparently minor, problems that their doctors suspect are diabetes-related, like repeated skin or other infections, such as boils or thrush (high blood glucose levels leave you more than usually susceptible to repeat infections). Other cases are found on routine examinations, say for life insurance, or at 'well woman' or 'well man' clinics. Some people are sent to their doctors by opticians, who have detected, on a routine test for glasses, early cataracts or changes in the retina (in the back of the eye) that point to diabetes.

Looking back afterwards, especially when they have started treatment for their diabetes and begin to feel better, such people usually realize that they have been 'under par'. However, most people like this have put their minor malaise down to their 'age' or 'stress', and are surprised by the diagnosis.

To Summarize

The classic symptoms of Type 2 diabetes are the gradual onset of thirst along with the need to pass more urine, day and night; tiredness, skin infections including thrush in the throat or in the vagina, in a person who is usually, but not always, overweight. However, because the symptoms have taken so long to develop fully, many people ignore them, or put them down to age and 'middle-aged spread'.

Partly because of this attitude, for every person in a developed country known to have Type 2 diabetes there is at least another with it who is yet to be diagnosed. In Britain, for example, that means that there are more than half a million known people with Type 2 diabetes, and another half million (at least) with the disease, but who do not know it. Just as important, neither do their doctors. Not only that, but half the people known to have Type 2 diabetes have no symptoms of it at all. They were diagnosed fortuitously when their urine was examined at a routine examination, and sometimes they resent having to be labelled with the disease and having to change their lives accordingly.

That resentment, though understandable, is misplaced and can even be dangerous if they deduce from their lack of symptoms that Type 2 diabetes is a mild disease and they need not change their lifestyle. It is a serious health problem that is just as likely to cause early death from heart attacks, strokes and kidney failure as Type 1 diabetes. Even if you feel well without treatment, you must keep it under strict control. If you do keep it under control, you can reduce your chances of an early heart attack, stroke or kidney failure by more than 50 per cent – and that is enormously worth your while.

How do you know you have your diabetes under control? In a very similar way to the instructions for people with Type 1 diabetes – by your blood glucose tests. They are used to make the diagnosis in the first place, and to judge your progress thereafter.

Making the Diagnosis

In the past, international organizations for the study of diabetes have disagreed on the details of how to make the diagnosis of Type 2 diabetes. The World Health Organization (WHO) advises that diabetes be diagnosed if the fasting plasma glucose (the first glucose level in the morning after a night without food) is more than 7.8 mmol/L, or a random plasma glucose level (a test taken at any time of day) is above 11.1 mmol/L. If the fasting plasma glucose is between 6.0 and 7.8 mmol/L, or the random plasma glucose is between 7.8 and 11.1 mmol/L, then an oral glucose tolerance test should be done. This involves swallowing 50 grams of glucose, with blood samples being taken two hours afterwards. If after two hours the plasma glucose is above 11.1 mmol/L, diabetes is diagnosed. If it is between 7.8 and 11.1 mmol/L, the patient has 'impaired glucose tolerance' – a halfway stage between normal and diabetes. If it is below 7.8 mmol/L, then the person is considered to be normal. People with fasting plasma glucose levels below 6 mmol/L, or random plasma glucose levels below 7.8 mmol/L, are considered not to have diabetes.

These rules were thought to be too cumbersome by the American Diabetes Association, which in 1997 advised its doctors to rethink how to diagnose Type 1 and Type 2 diabetes. The first was re-classified as Type 1 (beta-cell defect, usually auto-immune) and the second as Type 2 (insulin resistance with an insulin secretory defect). Type 2 was to be diagnosed entirely from a fasting plasma glucose level (taken first thing in the morning 12 hours after the last food) of 7.0 mmol/L or more. There were to be no oral glucose tolerance tests. If the fasting plasma glucose was between 6.0 and 7.0 mmol/L, then the patient was diagnosed as having impaired glucose tolerance. A fasting plasma glucose under 6.0 mmol/L meant no diabetes.

Several points should be made here. One is that plasma glucose (the amount of glucose in a blood sample after the red cells are removed) is the routine way that blood glucose levels are measured in laboratory machines, and is usually slightly higher than that in whole blood (which still contains the red cells). The other is that the difference between the Americans and WHO in the way the diagnosis is made has not yet been resolved. However, the American method saves a lot of time and cost, and will probably be adopted by most countries and specialists.

What this method also provides is a target at which every person with Type 2 diabetes can aim. If you can manage to keep your fasting plasma glucose under 7.0 mmol/L (this is equivalent to a finger-tip blood level of around 6 mmol/L), you are doing very well.

The reasons why you should take your diabetes team's advice very seriously is explained in the next chapter. Type 2 diabetes is hardly ever just about keeping your blood glucose in check: it is almost always part of a much more complex series of problems that is now labelled 'metabolic syndrome'. You must face up to every aspect of these problems if you wish to give yourself the best chance of surviving into a healthy old age. You could probably solve the problems set by your Type 2 diabetes by becoming a hunter-gatherer like your ancestors, but that might be socially unacceptable. Nevertheless, you can still do a lot for yourself by indulging in plenty of physical exercise and eating healthily. You may need medical help, too. The best way for doctors to provide this help is described in the next chapter, which describes the work of the United Kingdom Prospective Diabetes Study (UKPDS).

Chapter Nine

Type 2 Diabetes and the Metabolic Syndrome

Type 2 diabetes used to be thought of as the 'mild' form of the disease. After all, most people with it didn't have to take insulin injections. They didn't develop ketoacidosis, they didn't lapse into comas, and they were less likely to become blind or develop kidney failure than those with Type 1 diabetes. So as long as their blood glucose levels were reasonably controlled, it was assumed that they would sail on in life without much trouble. True, they did tend to have heart attacks and strokes a bit earlier in life than expected, but there was no proof that controlling their blood glucose more strictly would make any difference to that. And as most people with Type 2 diabetes felt reasonably well, there didn't seem much point in striving for better control, particularly as it might put them at risk of 'hypo' attacks (see page 32).

These attitudes to Type 2 diabetes started to change in the 1960s, largely as the result of work done by Professor Harry Keen, Professor of Human Metabolism, and his team at Guy's and St Thomas's Hospital in London. Professor Keen pointed out in the 1960s that there were 'bad companions' to diabetes – persistent high blood glucose levels, high blood pressure ('hypertension') and the appearance of microscopic amounts of protein in the urine, a sign of early kidney disease (microalbuminuria). All of these, he proposed, were mainly responsible for people with Type 2 diabetes dying early from strokes, heart attacks and kidney failure.

Professor Keen and his colleagues were far-sighted. It was largely as a result of their basic work on the long-term damage that Type 2 diabetes did to people that the United Kingdom Prospective Diabetes Study (UKPDS) was set up in the 1970s. The UKPDS made its reports in 1998, and it established not only the extent of the illnesses and deaths caused by Type 2 diabetes, but also how they could best be prevented.

On the way to these results, UKPDS added two more elements common to the cause of illness in Type 2 diabetes – abnormal blood lipid (cholesterol) levels, and smoking. In 1988, Dr G M Reaven named the combination of high blood glucose levels, high blood insulin levels, high blood pressure, high blood cholesterol levels and microalbuminuria as 'syndrome X'. He showed that people with this combination of problems had a very high risk of heart attack and stroke much earlier in life than would be normally expected, and suggested that all the factors that contributed to syndrome X be treated very vigorously to try to reduce that risk.

However, Professor Reaven's description was incomplete. One more illness-creating sign had to be added – central obesity. That is, people who were overweight in a particular way, who put on extra fat around their waists rather than round their buttocks and hips, and who possessed all the other syndrome X factors, too, were in particular danger. In effect, the apple-shaped person was at more risk than the pear-shaped!

The complete picture, combining all these signs and symptoms, is now known as 'metabolic syndrome'. UKPDS showed that most people with Type 2 diabetes have metabolic syndrome to some degree. In fact, their high blood pressure, abnormal blood lipids, their apple-shaped obesity, even their microalbuminuria were probably all present up to 10 years *before* they developed obvious Type 2 diabetes. Their 'signpost' to future diabetes would have been a slightly raised fasting blood plasma glucose level (between 6 and 7 mmol/L) and raised insulin levels. These figures are not enough to make the diagnosis of diabetes, but can be called 'pre-diabetic'. People in whom these results are found, especially if they are also overweight and have high blood pressure, must be treated exactly as if they already have diabetes. Their risk of strokes and heart attacks already rising – and should be minimized.

In effect, these people must keep their blood glucose, their blood pressure and their blood cholesterol levels under control. How this is done is what the rest of this book is about. It may sound complex, but really it isn't. You may even enjoy the challenge, and if you succeed you could well add 20 healthy and active years to your life expectancy.

UKPDS – Its Aims and Results

The best way to explain how to go about looking after yourself if you have Type 2 diabetes is to go over the aims and the results of the various UKPDS studies.

The first UKPDS study to be published (UKPDS 23, in the *British Medical Journal* on 14th March 1998) established beyond all doubt the extra health risks for people with Type 2 diabetes. The following studies, published later that year in the *British Medical Journal* and the *Lancet*, showed how the health risks could be vastly reduced by controlling blood glucose and blood pressure levels.

Before UKPDS 23 started, it had already been established that people with Type 2 diabetes were between two and three times more likely to have heart attacks and strokes than people of the same age without diabetes. The researchers also knew that when the people with diabetes had strokes and heart attacks, they were twice as likely to die from them as people not suffering from diabetes who'd had strokes and heart attacks of similar severity. So the main aim of UKPDS 23 was to find out why people with Type 2 diabetes were so susceptible to such early death.

Diabetes teams from all over the UK took part. The study followed 3,055 men and women with newly diagnosed Type 2 diabetes, but not, as yet, any symptoms or signs of heart disease, impending stroke, kidney disease or blindness, for an average of almost 8 years. During the study, 335 of them developed coronary artery disease, a much higher number than would have been expected in a similar group without diabetes (their average age was 52 years). Those who went on to develop heart disease had a higher HbA1c, higher blood pressure and higher fasting blood glucose levels, they smoked more and had smoked for longer, and they showed more abnormal blood cholesterol patterns than those who did not develop heart disease.

The researchers' conclusions left little room for argument. They wrote:

'A quintet of potentially modifiable risk factors for coronary artery disease exists in patients with Type 2 diabetes mellitus. These risk factors are increased concentrations of low density lipoprotein cholesterol, decreased concentrations of high density lipoprotein cholesterol, raised blood pressure, hyperglycaemia and smoking.'

Five more UKPDS study results followed UKPDS 23 in 1998. Two looked at better control of blood glucose levels, two at better control of high blood pressure, and one calculated the cost-effectiveness in controlling blood pressure better, in terms of savings in the treatment of serious heart disease.

UKPDS 33 (published in the *Lancet* on September 12th 1998, pages 837 to 853) followed 3,867 newly diagnosed people with Type 2 diabetes who after 3 months of diet alone still had high fasting plasma glucose levels (6.1 mmol/L or higher). They were allocated randomly either to 'conventional' treatment or 'intensive' treatment. The conventional treatment used diet alone to try to lower the fasting plasma glucose levels, and only used drugs if there were hyperglycaemic symptoms or the fasting plasma glucose level was above 15 mmol/L. The intensive treatment used drugs and insulin where necessary to keep the fasting blood glucose below 6 mmol/L.

After 10 years, the average HbA1c of the intensively treated group was 7.0 per cent, and of the conventional group, 7.9 per cent (both groups started with the same HbA1c). The intensively treated group had 12 per cent fewer 'diabetes-related endpoints' (complications brought on or contributed to by the diabetes) than the others, most being problems with the small blood vessels, such as the need for treatment of eye complications and deterioration in vision. This difference was considered on statistical analysis to be definitely due to the more intensive treatment.

There were 10 per cent fewer diabetes-related deaths, and 6 per cent fewer deaths from all causes, in the intensively treated group. The statistical rigour which had to be applied to these figures did not allow the authors to conclude that the more intensive treatment had caused the difference. It did allow them to conclude, however, that none of the drugs used (the sulphonylureas chlorpropamide, glibenclamide or glipazide) nor the insulin had made the risk of heart attacks and stroke worse.

UKPDS 34 concentrated on overweight patients with Type 2 diabetes (fewer than half of the patients in UKPDS 33 were overweight). It followed 753 people weighing at least 20 per cent more than their ideal weight who still had high fasting plasma glucose levels after 3 months of diet alone. As in UKPDS 33, the patients were split randomly into two groups, one of which continued to be treated conventionally, with diet alone, and the other intensively, with the drug metformin, aiming to keep their fasting plasma glucose level below 6 mmol/L. In a second analysis the results from the 342 patients given metformin were compared with those of 951 overweight patients treated intensively with a sulphonylurea in UKPDS 33. After 10.7 years, the metformin-treated group had an average HbA1c of 7.4 per cent, in contrast to the diet-only group's average of 8.0 per cent, so that the intensive group had been better controlled.

The results were quite definitive. There were 32 per cent fewer diabetes-related 'endpoints', 42 per cent fewer diabetes-related deaths, and 36 per cent fewer deaths from all causes in the metformin-treated group. Metformin had a better effect than the sulphonylureas on all endpoints in these overweight patients. The authors concluded:

'Since intensive glucose control with metformin appears to decrease the risk of diabetes-related endpoints in overweight diabetic patients, and is associated with less weight gain and fewer hypoglycaemic attacks than are insulin and sulphonylureas, it may be the first-line pharmacological therapy of choice in these patients.'

Put simply, both of these trials showed that intensive control of blood glucose levels in Type 2 diabetes helps avert complications like blindness and, if you are overweight, substantially reduces your chances of severe illness and death from heart attack, stroke and kidney disease.

Even these conclusions, however, are a little disappointing. Although better regulation of blood glucose levels did reduce the risks of illness and death, it did not reduce them enough. The two studies showed that we need more than 'good control' of glucose levels to lower them to a level approaching those in people who do not have diabetes.

UKPDS 38 and 39 offered an extra approach. They studied the effects of close blood pressure control in Type 2 diabetes. In UKPDS 38, 758 people with Type 2 diabetes with high blood pressure were allocated to what the doctors defined as 'tight' blood pressure control, and 390 patients to less tight control. The progress of both groups was followed for an average of 8.4 years.

Tight control meant bringing the blood pressure down to around 140/80 mm Hg, a figure accepted as being in the normal range. It meant persevering with higher doses and/or combinations of blood pressure-lowering (antihypertensive) drugs to drive the pressure down as far as possible in the 'tight control' group, and settling for standard doses of drugs in the less-controlled group. The tight control was successful in reducing the pressure – it brought the average blood pressure down from 160/94 to 144/82. Blood pressures in the group given less control fell from 160/94 to 154/87 – still an acceptable achievement under normal circumstances.

The results were very clear. Among the tight control patients there were 32 per cent fewer deaths due to the diabetes, 44 per cent fewer strokes, and 37 per cent fewer serious eye problems. By the end of the follow-up period, the group under tight blood pressure control had far better eyesight than those under less control, with far less deterioration in vision. However, to achieve the tight control, nearly a third (29 per cent) needed to take three or more different antihypertensive drugs. Although this was sometimes an inconvenience, it was rarely a problem. The authors of UKPDS 38 concluded: 'reducing blood pressure needs to have high priority in caring for patients with Type 2 diabetes.' They suggested that the minimum aim should be a blood pressure below 150/85 mm Hg.

UKPDS 39 was designed to compare the two main antihypertensive drugs (atenolol and captopril) used in the UKPDS 38 study: they both lowered the blood pressure to a similar extent, and they had similar beneficial effects. It was concluded that it was the lowering of the blood pressure itself, rather than any property of the individual drug, that protected the patients against heart attacks, strokes, kidney failure and failing eyesight.

In these days of scrupulous attention to health care costs, one further analysis of the UKPDS blood pressure studies is worth mentioning. Alastair Gray of the Health Economics Research Centre at Oxford University compared the extra costs to the NHS of the more intensive blood pressure control with what was saved by not having to care for the heart attacks, strokes, kidney failure and blindness that had been avoided. It came to £1,049 per year gained of life, or £434 per year if the costs were discounted at 6 per cent per year. He concluded:

'Tight control of blood pressure in hypertensive patients with Type 2 diabetes substantially reduced the cost of complications, increased the interval without complications, and survival, and had a cost effectiveness ratio that compares favourably with many accepted healthcare programmes.'

This has been a fairly complex chapter, but it has been necessary to show how important it is for you, if you have Type 2 diabetes, to follow the rules. If you want to keep as healthy as you can, and avoid deteriorating eyesight, the possibility of kidney failure and the probability of a heart attack or stroke, then you must keep strict control of both your blood glucose level and your blood pressure.

You must also not lose sight of the other risks – your cholesterol, your weight and, if you are mad enough to smoke, your smoking habit. The next few chapters will help you to control them, too.

Chapter Ten

Being in Control

If you have read this book from the beginning you will already have got the repeated message – you must be in control of your own life if you are to survive into a healthy old age. Let us assume that you have just been diagnosed as having Type 2 diabetes. How do we continue from this point?

The first thing is to find out how severe it is, and how many of the risk factors for metabolic syndrome you possess. That is done quickly and easily. You will be weighed and measured, and your waist measurement will be taken – so you will learn how obese you are, and what type of obesity it is.

Your blood pressure will be taken, as will your random blood glucose level, and a time will be arranged for you to return for a fasting blood glucose level. Just as important, you will have a blood lipid profile done, to check on those all-important LDL- and HDL-cholesterol levels, and your urine will be examined for microalbuminuria. Within a few days all the results will be back, and your doctor will have a plan of treatment to correct anything that needs correcting.

Getting the Weight Right – Eating Healthily

Let's take the different aspects of treatment one by one, starting with weight. If you are overweight, then you absolutely MUST lose ALL the extra pounds. This isn't the same advice on weight as is given to people who do not have diabetes but are overweight – most of them can be a few pounds over with no real risk attached. For you, being slim is a necessity. If you can lose those extra pounds, you may at the same time lose a lot of your other problems – your high blood pressure, your high blood glucose levels, your abnormal cholesterol profile, the lot. So go to it. Try to become that hunter-gatherer you really should be, at least in shape and energy, if not in lifestyle.

You know your height, so aim for a weight that brings your BMI (see the graph on page 50) into the middle range of normal – say 22.5. And be sensible in the way you go about it. You will surely have to abandon the eating habits that have made you overweight in the first place. The diabetes team looking after you is bound to have a dietician or a diabetes nurse trained in teaching healthy eating habits to people with diabetes. So make an appointment, and get learning.

The principles of what you must do are easy. You eat plenty of starchy carbohydrates and fibre, plenty of fresh fruit, moderate amounts of protein, and a minimum of fats, sugary foods and alcohol. You eat small meals regularly, rather than one or two large meals a day. For the fine details, however, you need to learn how to make meals appetizing, so that you actually *like* what you are eating and even enjoy preparing the food. For that, depend on the dietician for hints and ideas. He or she can advise on all sorts of different cuisines, including ethnic cooking, and tailor them to your needs.

Take family members along to the meeting with the dietician if you can, particularly if they are involved in cooking and preparing meals. It is just as important for them to know what you should be eating as it is for you. As everyone would benefit from the Type 2 diabetes style of eating, it will do them good if they eat along with you. It isn't easy to be the only one in the family eating healthily while the rest are stuffing themselves with beefburgers and chips, puddings, custard and ice creams.

I like to use the healthy eating 'pyramid' devised by Professor Paul Zimmet and Dr Matthew Cohen, of the International Diabetes Institute, Victoria, Australia, as a help to people wanting a quick check on what to eat most, what to eat in moderation, and what to eat least. It is reprinted here from the *Clinician's Manual on Non-Insulin Dependent Diabetes Mellitus*, published by Science Press in London.

People with Type 2 diabetes can be more flexible in their eating habits than those with Type 1, who need to correlate their eating with insulin injections. But they still need to eat their three meals a day, particularly if they are using hypoglycaemic drugs (about which more later). If you miss a meal while taking them you risk having a 'hypo'.

Frankly, losing weight successfully and staying in the BMI range of 20 to 25 is the most difficult instruction to follow for most people with Type 2 diabetes. Most feel hungry all the time, and find it very hard to change the eating habits of a lifetime. But you must do it. Remember that those very habits have been largely what has brought on your diabetes in the first place. So do persevere. You can do it, and you are not on your own. Your dietician and family and friends will support you if

Healthy Eating Pyramid

Eat least

Minimize fats, sugars and alcohol

Butter, margarine, cooking fat, oil, cream
Cakes, sweet biscuits, patries
Processed or fatty meat (e.g. bacon sausage, salami, pate)
Fried foods
Snack foods (e.g. chips, dips, nuts)
Chocolate
Ice cream
Mayonnaise, salad dressings
Confectionary
Soft drinks, cordial
Alcohol
Sugar
Honey
Jam
Jellies

Eat moderately

Have small servings of protein foods

Fish, seafood
Lean meat, skinless chicken
Eggs
Tofu
Cheese
Yoghurt
Milk

Eat most

Use these foods as the basis of every meal

Legumes and pulses (e.g. lentils, kidney beans, haricot beans)
Bread, especially pumpernickel or any bread with a large amount of grains
Breakfast cereals, preferably whole grain (especially rolled oats and bran)
Spaghetti and pasta
Fresh fruit, especially apples, pears, grapefuit, peaches, plums, oranges, cherries, firm bananas
Barley and rice
Vegetables, especially sweet potato, sweetcorn

you impress upon them how important it is for you.

How do you know if you are succeeding? Weigh yourself once a week, naked, on accurate bathroom scales at the same time of day and under the same circumstances (say, the same time after a meal). Measure round the widest part of your waist at the same time. Make a chart of both. And check your blood glucose level after different meals so that you learn which foods put it up more, and which ones less. If your attitude to these three simple actions is a good one, you will soon become enthusiastic about them and make progress. And as you do so, you will already be improving your blood glucose levels. After two or three months, you should even see your HbA1c (taken at your clinic visits) coming down.

Getting the Weight Right – Exercise

Eating correctly is only part of a weight-loss programme. The other part is exercise.

Exercise is at least as important as the correct eating habits for people with Type 2 diabetes – remember the hunter-gatherer theory? It is useful as a way of losing excess weight, but it is also especially useful as a direct aid to improving your sensitivity to insulin. The more exercise you do, the more efficient your muscles should become at taking up glucose and using it for energy, and the less you will need in the way of hypoglycaemic drugs or insulin. So just as becoming a normal weight is vital for you, so is the appropriate amount and type of exercise. You cannot afford to be a couch potato even if you are slim. You must exercise regularly, preferably at least three or four days a week.

This does not mean slavishly adhering to some pre-arranged programme of exercising. It is a very rare person who can keep that up for long – and for you, the change to regular exercise must be for life. So it must be the right exercise for you, in the right amount, and it must be safe.

In the past, doctors used to check the electrocardiograms of people with diabetes before advising them on the type of exercise they should do. This isn't considered quite so necessary as it was, as we have discovered that even people in heart failure can benefit from some exercise. But as people with Type 2 diabetes are more prone to heart problems, and circulation problems in the eyes, kidneys and legs, and difficulties with their peripheral nerves (neuropathy), it is advisable to choose your exercise carefully.

The first rule is that it isn't necessary for the exercise to be strenuous. Of course, if you like to run that's fine, but a brisk walk is good for you and any increase from your previous level of physical activity will be of benefit. It is important for the exercise to be of the aerobic type, in which you are taking in plenty of oxygen while exercising against very little resistance. Walking, cycling, swimming, even ballroom dancing are good examples. Aerobics classes are fine if you make sure first that you can cope with their length and range of activity, so find out what you are letting yourself in for first. Avoid step aerobics, as they put quite a lot of strain on the calf muscles and Achilles tendons: if you already have circulation problems, an injury may make them worse.

A good start is to exercise (a walk, for example) for 30 minutes a day, then increase the time and pace as you feel fitter. Once it becomes a bit more strenuous, warm up and warm down appropriately, finishing with a good stretch. As with your weight and waistline, have an exercise chart to keep you enthusiastic. And to prevent boredom, arrange to exercise with a friend, and to vary what you do from time to time.

One important point about exercise – wear the best possible shoes for the job. That goes without saying for people who don't have diabetes, but is particularly important for you, because you must keep your feet in good trim. The feet are often the weak spot in diabetes. The skin can so easily become infected, and they may be affected by poor circulation and by neuropathy, so that you don't notice when they are damaged. So take care of them – keep them clean and dry, with good nail care and free from athlete's foot, wear the proper socks (cotton, not nylon), and shoes that fit perfectly. Never compromise on shoes: they are the most important part of your clothing.

Alcohol and Smoking

If you think I have been strict with you so far on your lifestyle, wait until you have read this section. On alcohol, and particularly cigarettes, there should be no compromise. You must stick to moderate amounts of alcohol, if any at all. The advice is the same as for people with Type 1 diabetes (see page 49 for details): you must never drink on an empty stomach, you should stick to one or two standard drinks per day, and never binge.

As for smoking, you absolutely have to be a non-smoker, and avoid nicotine like the plague. If you can't do that, then there's little point in you reading on. Because any health advice you take will be nullified by your tobacco habit.

Why are doctors like myself so *severe* on tobacco? Because we are constantly having to deal with the human wreckage it causes, particularly when people have diabetes. Asked to devise a drug that attacks all the weak spots in diabetes, a mad scientist would only have to point to tobacco and its inhalation through the lungs. So if you are still a smoker and have diabetes of either type, Chapter Twelve is just for you. Non-smokers can miss it out!

Chapter Eleven

Keeping Glucose Levels Down

Managing your Type 2 diabetes has two main aims. One is to avoid and/or ease the symptoms of your diabetes, and the other is to prevent its long-term complications. We have established that the first is best achieved by keeping blood glucose levels as near normal as possible, and that the main way to do this is by eating healthily, taking plenty of exercise, losing any excess weight, drinking only moderately and not smoking at all.

Unfortunately, this ideal advice doesn't always work. You may find that, despite eating and exercising correctly and losing all your excess weight, your fasting blood glucose levels are still too high, and you still feel under par. Or you find that you can't manage to get your weight down enough, because you find it difficult to obey your new rules on eating and/or exercise. Either way, your new lifestyle has not brought your blood glucose levels into good enough control. Your doctor will then consider prescribing drugs that will help.

Such drugs are called 'oral hypoglycaemic agents'. They are swallowed as pills or capsules, and are NOT an alternative to, nor a substitute for, a better lifestyle. You must continue to eat healthily, exercise regularly and lose any excess weight while you are taking them. Occasionally they are prescribed soon after diagnosis of Type 2 diabetes, but only in cases thought to be relatively severe, with blood glucose levels above 17 mmol/L. As a routine they are started when healthy eating, exercise and weight loss have failed to bring glucose levels under control.

Hypoglycaemic agents are in three main groups – sulphonylureas, biguanides and alpha-glucosidase inhibitors. The chart below shows the hypoglycaemic agents in current use (in 2001).

In general, sulphonylureas are used for people of normal weight or who have been obese and have lost enough weight to show that they are conforming reasonably well with new lifestyle advice. Metformin (Glucophage), the single biguanide left on the market (others were abandoned because of side-effects), is the drug of choice for people who have been unable to lose enough weight, and who remain at least 20 per cent over their ideal weight (a BMI of 30 or more).

Hypoglycaemic agents:

Sulphonylureas:	Chlorpropamide	Diabinese
	Glibenclamide	Daonil, Euglucon
	Gliclazide	Amaryl
	Glipizide	Glibenese, Minodiab
	Gliquidone	Glurenorm
	Tolbutamide	Rastinon
Biguanides:	Metformin	Glucophage
Thiazolidinediones:	Pioglitazone	Actos
	Rosiglitazone	Avandia
Others:	Acarbose	Glucobay
	Repaglinide	NovoNorm

   Hypoglycaemic agents do bring down fasting and random glucose levels, but you must always continue to make regular checks on your blood glucose. If you are taking metformin, you also need regular checks on your kidney function. Oral hypoglycaemic agents are NOT useful for Type 1 diabetes, and are indeed never prescribed for it. If they do not prove to control Type 2 diabetes satisfactorily, despite increasing doses, trying another type of hypoglycaemic or combining them with other hypoglycaemics, then they should be stopped. Insulin may have to be used instead. There is no reason to use two different sulphonylureas together, but either the biguanide metformin or the alpha-glucosidase inhibitor acarbose may be added to a sulphonylurea if it has not adequately controlled the diabetes.

Sulphonylureas

Sulphonylureas probably act by inducing the pancreas to release more insulin, though on long-term treatment they may also reduce insulin resistance. The current sulphonylureas include glibenclamide (Daonil, Euglucon), gliclazide (Diamicron), glimepiride (Amaryl), and glipizide (Minodiab, Glibeneze). (Please note: where brand names are given they are UK ones; the brand names used in the US or other countries for these drugs may differ.)
   Sulphonylureas differ from each other in their potency and length of action, so that they vary in strength of dose and in the numbers of times

per day they should be taken. For example, glimepiride needs to be taken only once a day, while the others are usually given twice daily. Your diabetes specialist is probably best able to judge which one will suit you best, and may change the prescription after an initial assessment period, depending on the success of the results and how you feel on the drug.

All sulphonylureas can cause 'hypo' attacks, so you should be aware of this possibility and know about your particular early warning symptoms, such as sweating, shaking, palpitations, hunger, and perhaps pins and needles around the mouth. This is particularly true for older people, who may have very little in the way of hypo symptoms. Because of this, some diabetes specialists prefer not to prescribe sulphonylureas for the elderly.

If you are starting to have a hypo, immediately swallow the equivalent of 15 grams of glucose. That is, approximately one glass of lemonade or fruit juice, three heaped teaspoons of sugar, two barley sugars or five jelly beans. This can be repeated in five minutes if there is no obvious effect, and followed by a starchy meal (pasta, brown rice, wholegrain bread) to prevent a repeat attack. The sulphonylurea dose should be reduced and your treatment programme should be reviewed.

Some people mistake anxiety attacks for hypos – the symptoms may be superficially similar. A blood glucose test done during the attack should correct this mistake.

More serious than a mistaken anxiety attack is a hypo that comes on without any warning. This is labelled medically as 'hypoglycaemia unawareness' or 'asymptomatic hypoglycaemia'. It can happen to anyone treated with insulin or sulphonylureas, and the symptoms are the sudden onset of very peculiar behaviour or sudden loss of consciousness. The diagnosis is made from the low blood glucose reading taken with the patient's own kit, so it is advisable for people who are prone to such sudden hypos always to carry upon them their kit and instructions on what to do if they are found in such a state.

The treatment for hypoglycaemia is given on page 38, in the section on Type 1 diabetes, but it is worth repeating here because it is so crucial.

If someone is suffering from a 'hypo', do not try to pour liquid glucose into their mouth, as it may be inhaled and choke the patient. A smear of glucose gel or, failing that, honey, on the gums may help. The best treatment is an intravenous injection of dextrose, followed if necessary by a glucose drip. An alternative is an injection of a standard dose of glucagon deep into a muscle. Doctors carry glucose and glucagon in their emergency bags. A case could be made for the close relatives of some-one with frequent hypos like this to learn how to inject glucagon them-selves. However, adjustment of the sulphonylurea dose to avoid future attacks is a better way of dealing with them.

An increased appetite and the tendency to hypoglycaemia on sul-phonylureas give some people a tendency to moderate weight gain: they should be on guard against this becoming excessive. If you reach good blood glucose control on a sulphonylurea, then you should con-sider reducing the dose or doing without it altogether, particularly if you are overweight.

Sulphonylurea side-effects are few, the most common being mild indigestion or gastric upsets.

It used to be recommended that sulphonylureas be given 30 minutes before meals. Now it is accepted that they can be taken during meals. They may interfere with the action of the anticoagulant drug warfarin (a treatment to prevent thromboses after heart attacks, strokes and heart surgery), so these drugs are not usually given together. People taking warfarin are usually prescribed metformin and/or acarbose instead.

Biguanides

The biguanide metformin (Glucophage) delays the absorption of glu-cose from the gut into the bloodstream, interferes with the production of glucose from glycogen and fat stores in the liver, and increases the uptake of glucose from the bloodstream into the tissues. It therefore has three beneficial actions in Type 2 diabetes. It is usually given as the drug of first choice for Type 2 diabetes in people who remain 20 per cent or more overweight. It can also be given with a sulphonylurea or with acarbose, as the different effects of the three types of drug are complementary.

Metformin is given twice a day, usually starting at a dose of 500 mg. The maximum dose is 1 gram twice daily. Its common side-effects include loss of appetite, nausea and diarrhoea, which occur in around 1 in 12 patients (8 per cent). However, the mild loss of appetite may even be useful for most patients, considering they are usually over-weight in the first place. Less common is a metallic taste in the mouth, and an anaemia related to its interference with vitamin B12 absorp-tion. An advantage of metformin is that its reduction of blood glucose levels is never enough to cause a 'hypo' attack when prescribed on its own. It should be given with or after meals to avoid stomach upsets.

A very rare side-effect of metformin is 'lactic acidosis'. This is a life-threatening emergency in which the patient becomes suddenly very ill. However, it is virtually confined to the very old, to people with kidney or liver disease, or to those who are in heart failure or have severe peripheral vascular disease (such as pre-gangrenous changes in the feet). So people who are at risk of lactic acidosis from metformin are usually on a close watch for the early signs of the condition. Lactic acidosis was the reason for the withdrawal of a previous biguanide, phenformin, from the market. At the time, metformin was shown to be much less likely to cause it.

Acarbose

Acarbose (Glucobay), an alpha-glucosidase inhibitor, is one of a kind. It acts by delaying the digestion of sugars into glucose in the gut, so that the rise in blood glucose after a meal is much slower than usual and reaches a lower peak. Because of this action, acarbose also reduces the amount of insulin produced by the pancreas in response to a meal, so that it not only reduces blood glucose levels, it also reduces the high blood insulin levels in people with early Type 2 diabetes. Trials have shown that acarbose also reduces HbA1c levels to a moderate degree (say from 9 to 8 per cent). It is given either alone or along with a sulphonylurea or metformin.

Started at a low dose which is gradually increased, the main side-effects of acarbose, diarrhoea and wind, can be kept to a minimum. They usually subside if the treatment is continued, especially if you avoid eating foods containing simple sugars like glucose and sucrose. Most people start on 50 mg three times a day, then gradually increase it to 100 mg or, less often, 200 mg.

The Glitazones: Rosiglitazone and Pioglitazone

The Glitazones, Rosiglitazone and Pioglitazones, were introduced into Britain in 2000/2001 as a development onwards from the sulphonylureas. Classified as a 'thiazolidinediones', they reduce blood glucose levels by reducing insulin resistance in fatty tissues, muscles and the liver. In theory, therefore, it is correcting the defect specific to Type 2 diabetes. At the time of writing they only have a licence for use as a second agent to be given along with metformin in obese patients for whom metformin alone has not produced satisfactory diabetes control. Alternatively, it is given with a sulphonylurea in patients who cannot tolerate metformin or who cannot have metformin for other reasons (such as warfarin therapy).

Glitazones can be taken once or twice daily, with or without food. Their main problem is that they can cause or make worse fluid retention; this can induce heart failure in susceptible patients. They also need to be monitored regularly for liver problems, as there have been a few reports that it may cause jaundice. This can be avoided if blood tests are taken for 'liver enzymes', a rise in which is an early sign of a liver reaction. If the drug is stopped at this point, the reaction will reverse and no harm will be done. The advantage of adding glitazones to either a sulphonylurea or metformin is much better blood glucose control.

Repaglinide (Novonorm)
Repaglinide is a drug unrelated to any of the other glucose lowering medicines that acts by stimulating the release of insulin from the pancreas. It is taken before each main meal, so that its action, which is short, occurs only when blood glucose levels are highest, and it has no effect by the time they have returned to normal. Theoretically it should not cause hypoglycaemia when taken in this way.

The Time for Insulin

If, despite the change in your eating habits, the extra exercise, weight loss and the use of sulphonylureas, metformin, acarbose and rosiglitazone, you still can't get your blood glucose under control, you may have to start on insulin injections.

Your doctor will first of all try to find out why the attempts at good control have failed. The most common cause is failure to stick to the correct eating pattern. If this is due to a misunderstanding about what you should be eating or why you should be eating it, then reading this book should help. Failure to take the tablets regularly is the second most common cause of poor diabetes control. Do try to follow the instructions. Go to the extent of having a small alarm on your watch if necessary, to remind you of the pill-taking time each day.

Emotional stress is yet another cause of poor control. It may cause you to revert back to your old lifestyle – eating badly, drinking more, going back to cigarettes. Or the extra adrenaline and anxiety may have a direct effect on your glucose levels. So recognize the times when you may need to monitor your glucose levels more closely, and act upon them. And get advice about how to manage your stress from the appropriate person in your professional diabetes team.

Illnesses such as infections (like severe influenza, gastroenteritis or a urinary infection) and an overactive thyroid ('thyrotoxicosis') may cause you to lose your blood glucose control. If so, the correct action is to get help urgently: this is no time to increase doses of, or change, your hypoglycaemic agent. It is much safer to go on insulin for a while until the illness is brought under control. Your diabetes team will give you very detailed advice on how to do this.

There are a few people with newly diagnosed Type 2 diabetes whose blood glucose fails to respond to any of the oral hypoglycaemic agents. This is called 'primary failure of oral treatment': such people need to be put on insulin permanently. Insulin may be needed, too, in the very small number of people with Type 2 diabetes who lose their control for no obvious reason after having managed it well for years with hypogly-caemic agents. This is known as 'secondary failure'. Many primary and secondary failure patients actually may have an unusual form of Type 1 diabetes that develops slowly after an onset that seems like the Type 2 disease.

If you have Type 2 diabetes that has begun to need insulin, and infection, thyroid disease or severe stress have been ruled out, then you should consider yourself as a Type 1 patient and organize your life accordingly. The first half of this book explains how best to do this.

Most people who have to go on to insulin after oral treatment manage well on a single dose of long-acting insulin per day, and can combine it with a hypoglycaemic agent. The transition period on to insulin is usually managed with the patient being a day patient at the diabetes centre or clinic, or even by visits to the home, each morning until the control is adequate. As with Type 1 diabetes, the insulin dose is adjusted according to the blood glucose levels. It is best to keep the insulin dose as low as possible, as higher doses (say more than 50 units per day) will raise blood insulin levels, which could make your metabolic syndrome worse by tending to raise blood pressure and worsening the blood cho-lesterol profile.

As the UKPDS studies showed, it is vital to manage blood pressure and blood cholesterol levels as well as possible, on top of getting the glucose control right. How this is done is the subject of Chapter Thir-teen.

'Good' and 'Bad' Glucose Control

You may be wondering, however, before you read on, what actually is 'good' and what is 'bad' glucose control. With Type 2 diabetes, you should be doing pre- and post-meal blood glucose tests once or twice a week, even if you are well controlled. If the control is less than good, or you are changing your treatment, you need to test more often.

The ideal fasting and after-meal blood glucose levels are, respectively, under 6 mmol/L and under 8 mmol/L. They go with an HbA1c under 7 per cent and no glucose in the urine test. We accept as 'good' control pre-meal and post-meal blood glucose levels, respectively, of under 8 mmol/L and under 11 mmol/L, and an HbA1c between 7 and 7.9 per cent. Levels above these are considered to range from fair control to poor control (this last defined as pre-meal and post-meal blood glucose levels above 10 and above 13 mmol/L respectively, with more than one 'plus' of glucose in the urine and an HbA1c of more than 9 per cent).

If you are not in the good or ideal group, then you need to do much better, and to review all aspects of your lifestyle, weight and treatment. If you leave yourself in the fair or poor control group, you face very high risks. There are always ways to improve, and you should be very serious about doing so.

Part Four
Complications

Chapter Twelve

Why You Mustn't Smoke –
And How to Stop If You Do

Smoking is a stupid, suicidal habit for anyone, no matter how healthy. It is even worse, if that is possible, for people with diabetes, because it multiplies all the extra risks they face of heart disease, strokes and kidney disease. So if you are a smoker, you must be a non-smoker before you put this book down.

How, exactly, does smoking harm you? Tobacco smoke contains carbon monoxide and nicotine. The first poisons the red blood cells, so that they cannot pick up and distribute much-needed oxygen to the organs and tissues, including the heart muscle. Carbon monoxide-affected red cells (in the 20-a-day smoker, nearly 20 per cent of red cells are carrying carbon monoxide instead of oxygen) are also stiffer than normal, so that they can't bend and flex through the smallest blood vessels. The gas also directly poisons the heart muscle, so that it cannot contract properly and efficiently, thereby delivering a 'double whammy' of damage which a diabetic heart, already working under the disadvantage of high blood glucose and high blood pressure, can ill afford.

Nicotine causes small arteries to narrow, so that the blood flow through them slows. It raises blood glucose levels and blood cholesterol levels, thickening the blood and promoting the degenerative process in the artery walls – which is already faster than normal in diabetes. Both nicotine and carbon monoxide encourage the blood to clot, multiplying the risks of coronary thrombosis and a thrombotic stroke.

Add to all this the tars that smoke deposits in the lungs, which further reduce the ability of red cells to pick up oxygen, and the scars and damage to the lungs that always in the end produce chronic bronchitis and sometimes induce cancer, and you have a formula for disaster.

Here are the bald facts about smoking. If they do not convince you to stop, then you may as well give up reading this book, because there is no point in being 'health conscious' if you continue to indulge in tobacco. Its ill effects will counterbalance any good that your doctors can do for you.

Smoking causes more deaths from heart attacks than from lung cancer and bronchitis.

People who smoke are two or three times more likely to have a fatal heart attack than non-smokers. The risk rises with rising numbers of cigarettes smoked, and is doubled if you also have diabetes.

Men under 45 who smoke 25 or more cigarettes a day have a 10- to 15-times greater chance of death from heart attack than non-smoking men of the same age.

About 40 per cent of all heavy smokers, even if they do not have diabetes, die before they reach 65. Of those who reach that age, many are disabled by bronchitis, angina, heart failure and leg amputations, all because they smoked. Diabetes makes all these risks of smoking much greater. Only 10 per cent of smokers survive in reasonable health to the age of 75. Most non-smokers reach 75 in good health.

In Britain, 40 per cent of all cancer deaths are from lung cancer, which is very rare in non-smokers. Of 441 British male doctors who died from lung cancer, only seven had never smoked. Only one non-smoker in 60 develops lung cancer; the figure for heavy smokers is one in six!

Other cancers more common in smokers than in non-smokers include tongue, throat, larynx, pancreatic, kidney, bladder and cervical cancers.

The very fact that you are reading this book means that you are taking an intelligent interest in your health. So after reading so far, it should be common sense to you not to smoke. Yet it is very difficult to stop, and many people who need an excuse for not stopping put up spurious arguments for their stance. Here are ones that every doctor is tired of hearing, and my replies:

My father/grandfather smoked 20 a day and lived till he was 75.

Everyone knows someone like that, but they conveniently forget the many others they have known who died long before their time. The chances are that you will be one of them, rather than one of the lucky few.

People who don't smoke also have heart attacks.

True. There are other causes of heart attacks, but 70 per cent of all people under 65 admitted to coronary care with heart attacks are smokers, as are 91 per cent of people with angina considered for coronary bypass surgery.

I believe in moderation in all things, and I only smoke moderately.

That's rubbish. We don't accept moderation in mugging, or dangerous driving, or exposure to asbestos (which, incidentally, causes far fewer deaths from lung cancer than smoking). Younger men who are only moderate smokers have a much higher risk of heart attack than non-smoking men of the same age. The figures are even worse for women with diabetes, who have a higher risk of heart attack than women of the same age who do not have diabetes.

I can cut down on cigarettes, but I can't stop.

It won't do you much good if you do. People who cut down usually inhale more from each cigarette and leave a smaller butt, so that they end up with the same blood levels of nicotine and carbon monoxide. You must stop completely.

I'm just as likely to be run over in the road as to die from my smoking.

In Britain, about 15 people die on the roads each day. This contrasts with 100 deaths a day from lung cancer, 100 from chronic bronchitis and 100 from heart attacks, almost all of which are due to smoking. Of every 1,000 young men who smoke, on average one will be murdered, six will die on the roads, and 250 will die from their smoking habit. Those risks increase for men and women with diabetes.

I have to die from something.

In my experience this is always said by someone in good health. They no longer say it after their heart attack or stroke, or after they have coughed up blood.

I don't want to be old, anyway.

We define 'old' differently as we grow older. Most of us would like to live a long time, without the inconvenience of being old. If we take care of ourselves on the way to becoming old we have at least laid the foundations for enjoying our old age.

I'd rather die of a heart attack than something else.

Most of us would like a fast, sudden death, but many heart attack victims leave a grieving partner in their early 50s to face 30 years of loneliness. Is that really what you wish?

Stress, not smoking, is the main cause of heart attacks.

Not true. Stress is very difficult to measure and very difficult to relate to heart attack rates. In any case, you have to cope with stress, whether you smoke or not. Smoking is an extra burden that can never help, and it does not relieve stress. It isn't burning the candle at both ends that causes harm, but burning the cigarette at one end.

I'll stop when I start to feel ill.

That would be fine if the first sign of illness were not a full-blown heart attack from which more than a third die in the first four hours.

It's too late to stop then.

I'll put on weight if I stop smoking.

You probably will, because your appetite will return and you will be able to taste food again. But if you follow the advice given in the section in this book about changing your eating habits to control your diabetes better, then you will lose any extra weight anyway. In any case, the benefits of stopping smoking far outweigh the few extra pounds you may put on.

I enjoy smoking and don't want to give it up.

Is that really true? Is that not just an excuse because you can't stop? Ask yourself what your real pleasure is in smoking, and try to be honest with the answer.

Cigarettes settle my nerves. If I stopped I'd have to take a tranquillizer.

Smoking is a prop, like a baby's dummy, but it solves nothing. It doesn't remove any causes of stress, and only makes things worse because it adds a promoter of bad health. And when you start to have symptoms, like the regular morning cough, it only makes you worry more. It will also make it more difficult for you to control your diabetes.

I'll change to a pipe or cigars – they are safer.

Lifelong pipe and cigar smokers are less prone than cigarette smokers to heart attacks, but have five times the risk of lung cancer and 10 times the risk of chronic bronchitis that non-smokers have. Again, double these figures for people with diabetes. Cigarette smokers who switch to pipes or cigars continue to be at high risk of heart attack, probably because they inhale.

I've been smoking now for 30 years – it's too late to stop now.

It's not too late, whenever you stop. The risk of sudden death from a first heart attack falls away very quickly after stopping, even after a lifetime of smoking. If you stop after surviving a heart attack, then you halve the risk of a second. It takes longer to reduce your risk of lung cancer, but it falls by 80 per cent over the next 15 years, no matter how long you have been a smoker.

I wish I could stop. I've tried everything, but nothing has worked.

Stopping smoking isn't easy unless you really want to do it. You have to make the effort yourself, rather than think that someone else can do it for you. So you must be motivated. If the next few pages do not motivate you, then nothing will.

You must find the right reason for yourself to stop. For someone with diabetes it should surely include that your diabetes will be under much better control, and you will be giving yourself a much better chance of remaining healthy for much longer. But there are plenty of other reasons.

For teenagers, who see middle-age and sickness as remote possibilities, and who see smoking as exciting and dangerous, the best attacks on smoking are the way it makes them look and smell. You can also add the environmental pollution of cigarette ends and the way big business exploits Third World nations, keeping their populations in poverty while they make huge profits by using land that should be used for growing food to cultivate tobacco. Pakistan uses 120,000 acres, and Brazil half a million acres of their richest agricultural land to grow tobacco. And as the multinationals are now promoting their product very heavily to the developing world, no teenager who smokes can claim to be really concerned about the health of the Third World. This is often as persuasive an argument in persuading a teenager to stop (or not to start) as any about health or looks.

For some older women, the key may be looks. Smoking ages people prematurely, causing wrinkles and giving a pale, pasty complexion. Women smokers experience the menopause at an earlier age, even in their mid-thirties, which can destroy the plans of businesswomen to have their families after a shot at a career.

For most men and women, the prime motivation is better health. The statistics for men and women in their 60s who smoke but do not have diabetes are frightening enough, without bringing in diabetes to further worsen them. More than a third of smoking men fail to reach pension age – add many more to that figure if they also have diabetes of either type.

Let us assume you are now fully motivated. How do you stop? It is easy. You become a non-smoker, as if you have never smoked. You throw away all your cigarettes and decide never to buy or accept another one. Announce the fact to all your friends, who will usually support you, and that's that. Most people find that they don't have true withdrawal symptoms, provided they are happy to stop. A few become agitated, irritable, nervous, and can't sleep at night. But people who have had to stop for medical reasons, say because they have been admitted to coronary care, hardly ever have withdrawal symptoms.

This strongly suggests that the symptoms are psychological rather than physical. And if you are stopping because you have found you have diabetes, that is not too different from the coronary care scenario. If you can last a week or two without a smoke, you will probably never light up again. The desire to smoke will disappear as the levels of carbon monoxide, nicotine and tarry chemicals in your lungs, blood, brain and other organs gradually subside.

If you must stop gradually, plan ahead. Write down a diary of the cigarettes you will have, leaving out one or two each succeeding day, and stick to it. Carry nicotine chewing gum or get a patch if you must, but remember that the nicotine is still harmful. Don't look on it as a long-term alternative to a smoke. If you are having real difficulty stopping, ask your doctor for a prescription of Zyban. You may be offered a two-month course of the drug. It helps, but is by no means infallible.

If you do use some kind of outside help to stop (others include acupuncture and hypnosis), remember they have no magical properties. They are a crutch to lean on while you make the determined effort to stop altogether. They cannot help if your will to stop is weak.

Recognize, too, that stopping smoking is not an end in itself. It is only part of your new way of life, which includes your new way of eating and exercise, and your new attitude to your future health. And you owe it not only to yourself but also to your partner, family and friends, because it will help to give them a healthier you for, hopefully, years to come. You are not on your own. More than a million Britons have stopped smoking each year for the last 15 years. Only one in three adults now smokes (fewer than one in 20 doctors). By stopping you are joining the sensible majority.

ChapterThirteen

Keeping Complications at Bay

As mentioned at the beginning of Chapter Eleven, every diabetic has two aims. The first, to keep blood glucose levels as near normal as possible, was dealt with in that chapter. The second, how to keep the complications of the diseases at bay, is dealt with in this chapter. It applies as much to people with Type 1 diabetes as to those with Type 2 disease.

The UKPDS studies described in Chapter Nine proved that keeping blood pressure down is vital to preventing the heart attacks, strokes, kidney disease, blindness and peripheral vascular disease (which leads to amputations) that plague people with both types of diabetes. There is plenty of other evidence from studies of the link between blood cholesterol levels and heart disease, which affects many people with Type 2 diabetes, that correcting abnormal blood cholesterol levels is just as important.

Of course, eating healthily and exercising regularly can bring the blood pressure down and go a long way to correcting the cholesterol profile, but for many people these measures are not enough. Their blood pressure remains too high, and the cholesterol levels remain wrong. They need help from antihypertensive (blood pressure-lowering) and hypolipidaemic (cholesterol-lowering) drugs.

Antihypertensive Drugs

Learning about antihypertensive drugs is as easy as A, B, C, D: A stands for ACE-inhibitors, B for beta-blockers, C for calcium-antagonists, and D for diuretics. They all lower blood pressure by different mechanisms, so that if one does not hit the target blood pressure for you, it can be combined with one or two of the others. Combinations of drugs almost always finally bring the blood pressure down into the area that gives the least risk of heart attack, stroke, kidney failure, blindness and amputation for peripheral circulation problems.

Until the UKPDS results, many experts in diabetes preferred to choose the ACE-inhibitors and calcium-antagonists over the beta-blockers and diuretics as their first choice, because of fears that the beta-blockers and diuretics might make the metabolic syndrome worse (by worsening the glucose and lipid profiles). However, UKPDS compared the beta-blocker atenolol with the ACE-inhibitor captopril, and the drugs were equally effective. The conclusion was that the important factor in reducing long-term risks was the lowering of the blood pressure itself, and not the type of drug that reduced it.

One rule about the choice of antihypertensive agent still stands, however. If there is any evidence of kidney disease (such as microalbuminuria), then an ACE-inhibitor, which has properties that protect the kidneys, is the drug of first choice.

The aim of all high blood pressure treatment is to bring blood pressure down into the normal range. For diabetes of either type this means a figure below 130/80 if possible, and certainly below 140/90. A detailed explanation of how these figures are arrived at is outside the remit of this book, but if you wish to know more, please see another book I have written, *Living with High Blood Pressure* (Sheldon Press, 2001), in which the latest guidelines of the International Hypertension Society are reported.

Your diabetes team will favour for their patients a particular group of drugs and drug combinations in which they have special expertise, and will choose the drug or drugs they consider to be most suitable for you. What is important is not the drug you are taking, but how effective it is at bringing down, and keeping down, your blood pressure. If the first drugs do not achieve the target blood pressure, the doses may be raised or other drugs may be added. Your diabetes team will be following strict guidelines on when and how to raise the doses or add new drugs, so be patient. It may take several months to gain full control, but the vast majority achieve it in the end.

When taking your antihypertensive tablets, please follow the instructions carefully. Keep in mind that your blood pressure control is just as important as your blood glucose control in helping you avoid heart attacks, strokes, blindness, kidney failure and amputations in the future. You cannot tell from how you feel whether your blood pressure is high or low. The only way to know is by measuring it, so this has to be done weekly for a while until it is stable, then at least monthly after that. Never miss your blood pressure appointment.

Controlling Cholesterol

How the lipids (fats) in the blood affect your risk of future heart attacks and strokes is a complex subject that needs another whole book for a detailed explanation. It is enough to say here that fats in the blood are carried around the body linked to proteins called lipoproteins. Cholesterol is a fat, so that it is transported as a cholesterol-lipoprotein. Cholesterol-lipoprotein combinations are classified according to their physical structure, which makes a difference to the density (basically the 'hardness' or 'softness') of the fatty globules that float in your bloodstream. They therefore may be high-density lipoprotein-cholesterol (HDL-C), or low-density lipoprotein-cholesterol (LDL-C). Other types included in routine laboratory analysis are very-low-density and intermediate-density lipoprotein-cholesterols, or VLDL and IDL. A person's total cholesterol level is simply the sum of them all.

Fat is also transported around the body as triglycerides (TG), and levels of these are also measured to provide your health care team with useful information.

Put simply (the story is a bit more complex than explained here, but this is a practical system which can be used to determine risk of heart disease), LDL-C and TG are the 'bad' lipids, and HDL-C is the 'good' lipid. LDL-C and TG are involved in *depositing* fats into artery walls, HDL-C *removes* the fatty material from the arteries.

So a high LDL-C and TG, with a low HDL-C, is a bad pattern of lipids which increases your risk of heart attacks and strokes. Make the LDL-C and TG lower and the HDL-C higher and you reduce the risk of heart attack and stroke. This is precisely the aim of lipid-lowering drugs. Many trials in many thousands of people with and without diabetes have shown that lowering total cholesterol levels (most cholesterol is in the form of LDL-C, so that generally lowering cholesterol will lower LDL-C the most) cuts deaths from heart attacks and strokes by around 30 to 40 per cent.

When you have your blood cholesterol checked, the total cholesterol is often the figure used to see how much you are at risk. Any total cholesterol figure above 5.5 mmol/L is considered high, and needs treatment. The usual treatment is advice on lifestyle changes (healthier eating and more exercise); if these steps do not succeed, cholesterol-lowering drugs are considered if the total cholesterol figure remains above 6 mmol/L.

If you have Type 2 diabetes, the relatively easy-going advice given to most people who do not have diabetes is not nearly enough. If your lipid levels are high, you have a greater need to reduce them because your chances of having heart attacks and strokes are so much higher than in the average population.

The standard target for people with diabetes is a total cholesterol below 5 mmol/L, and triglyceride (TG) levels below 2 mmol/L. TG is important, as it tends to be much higher than normal in people with Type 2 diabetes, and is usually linked to low HDL-C levels. The two measurements – high TG and low HDL-C together – add considerably to your risk of heart disease and stroke. It's worth noting that these can be present without the total cholesterol level being abnormally high.

So, for people with Type 2 diabetes the total cholesterol level may not be raised, but their TG and HDL-C levels may be such that they need treatment. This is why many diabetes clinics now treat on the basis of a 'lipid profile' which measures all the different forms of cholesterol, including TG, and not just total cholesterol alone.

Of particular importance is that the lipid abnormalities (in TG and HDL-C especially) in Type 2 diabetes often appear long before the diagnosis of the diabetes itself. People with Type 2 diabetes face two to four times the risk of coronary heart disease of people without diabetes, an excess related more to the lipid problem than to the high blood glucose or even the high blood pressure. Treating the lipid abnormalities in diabetes is therefore extremely important.

Hypoglycaemic agents such as the sulphonylureas and metformin reduce TG levels a little, but have no significant effect on other lipids. Increasing exercise and losing weight do lower TG and raise HDL-C, but not necessarily to the required levels. Many people with Type 2 diabetes need drugs to complete the job.

Statins and Fibrates

The choice of drugs to correct the lipids lies between 'statins' and 'fibrates'. They both lower LDL-C and TG levels and raise HDL-C. The current tendency is to use fibrates to lower excessively high TG, and to use statins to lower LDL-C. Some patients may need both: they can be taken together. The choice of drug depends largely on your lipid profile, and the experience of the diabetes team in handling the different drugs. There are five statins and four fibrates on the market in 2001. They differ in their details, but only slightly in their effects on blood lipids. It is now clear that they not only change lipid profiles towards a pattern linked to far fewer heart attacks and strokes, but their use actually reduces the numbers of heart attacks and strokes by between a third and a half.

A last point about lipid levels. Some people have raised triglyceride (TG) levels, but their HDL-C and LDL-C levels are in the normal range. This pattern is mostly caused by overindulgence in alcohol, so do not be surprised or annoyed if your doctor, faced with these results, suggests that you cut down severely on your drinking.

Chapter Fourteen

'Microvascular' Complications

Until now, this book has been all about how to prevent the complications of diabetes, but has not spelled out in detail what these complications are. Throughout the book there has been a repeated theme. People with diabetes of either type hardly ever die nowadays from the immediate consequences of poor glucose control, but they do die early from strokes, heart attacks and kidney failure, and they go blind, suffer nerve problems, and have circulation problems needing, sometimes, amputations.

This chapter reviews how these complications happen, and how, when they do happen, they can be treated.

I have divided the complications of diabetes into 'microvascular' and 'macrovascular' events. In microvascular complications, the smallest blood vessels in the body become thickened, narrowed and fragile, so that it is very easy for the blood to clot within them, blocking off the circulation beyond the clot, or for bleeds to occur from them, damaging the tissues immediately around the bleed.

Microvascular disease is especially damaging to two organs: the eyes and the kidneys. In the eyes this is called *retinopathy*, and in the kidneys it is called *nephropathy*. Microvascular disease also affects the nerves to the limbs, so that the brain receives the wrong messages from the nerves. This is known as *peripheral neuropathy*.

Diabetic Retinopathy

Diabetic retinopathy can be diagnosed and followed up by using an ophthalmoscope to look at the retina. Instead of the usual network of clearly defined blood vessels against a smooth pink background, the doctor will see small 'aneurysms' (like tiny red blobs) on or beside the blood vessels. There may be smudges of red which represent bleeds, and paler 'exudates', often like bits of cotton wool, which are areas of leakage of fluids into the tissues. Repeated eye examinations will show whether the condition is worsening, stabilizing or even improving with treatment. If it does become much worse, extensive laying down of new blood vessels inside the eye and deterioration in the centre of the retina leads to blindness.

Early retinopathy is seen in a quarter of people with Type 2 diabetes on the day they are diagnosed, so the process has started long before the diabetes itself is obvious. Within 8 years of diagnosis, half of all people with diabetes show some retinopathy, and after 20 years almost every person with diabetes shows some signs of it. This should not depress you. Nowadays very few people with Type 1 or Type 2 diabetes become blind, because those with early retinopathy are followed very closely, and impending trouble can usually be prevented by new techniques such as laser treatment to deal with those new blood vessels and bleeding points.

So if you have been told you have some signs of retinopathy, don't worry about it. But do be very strict about your eye tests. Everyone with diabetes must have an annual eye examination, and go for more frequent tests if they find that their vision is worsening. If retinopathy is diagnosed, it is usual to have a test every six months or more often, depending on its severity and progression.

During the test for retinopathy you will also be checked for early signs of cataract development. Cataracts are also a common complication of diabetes of either type. New techniques to replace cataracts with artificial lenses are a vast improvement on the old, and have greatly improved the outlook for people with diabetes who, a generation ago, would have been left virtually blind by this condition.

It can't be stressed enough that if you have retinopathy you can do a lot for yourself by keeping your blood glucose levels under very tight control. The huge US Diabetes Control and Complication Trial (DCCT) proved beyond all doubt that good control delayed the start and slowed the progression of all three microvascular complications – retinopathy, nephropathy and neuropathy. Reducing HbA1c levels from 9 to 7 per cent (proof of good control) reduced the risks of all three by a massive 60 per cent. So if you have been diagnosed as having any of these complications, you have an extra incentive to control your diabetes better.

Diabetic Nephropathy

Like retinopathy, diabetic nephropathy starts to affect the kidney before the diabetes itself is recognized. For many years it causes no noticeable symptoms at all, but it is easily detectable because the microscopic changes in the affected kidneys cause them to 'leak' tiny amounts of protein into the urine. This is picked up on a routine urine test for 'microalbuminuria'.

The detection of anything over 30 mg of protein in a litre (30 mg/L) of urine is defined as microalbuminuria. It means that you are at risk of future kidney disease, and also at particular risk of the 'macrovascular' complications of heart attacks and strokes.

The natural history of microalbuminuria is for it to worsen over the years. Eventually enough protein is leaked into the urine for it to be detected by a normal protein 'dipstick' test (which is at least a 10-fold increase on the microalbuminuria level). From that point it is only a matter of about seven years to complete kidney failure, needing dialysis and transplant.

Happily this progression can be stopped with excellent control of both blood glucose and high blood pressure. The aim for everyone with microalbuminuria is to have a blood pressure of around 120/80 or even lower. There is good evidence that this greatly improves their long-term outlook, in particular helping them to avoid eventual kidney failure. The blood pressure will probably fall somewhat with good glucose control and regular exercise anyway, but many experts now recommend that ACE-inhibitors be used, too, not just because they bring down the pressure further, but also because they seem specifically to protect the kidneys against further deterioration.

Once you have been found to have microalbuminuria, you must have regular blood tests to check your kidney function for the rest of your life. They will show if and how fast your kidneys are deteriorating, and be a guide on how best to manage it. Never miss your kidney tests. They are vital to your future.

Diabetic Neuropathy

Diabetic neuropathy usually takes the form of loss of the ability to sense pain and temperature in a 'stocking and glove' pattern, starting first in the feet, then spreading to the hands. Other symptoms include numbness, a burning sensation and feelings of pins and needles, which start in the toes and fingers and spread into the hands and feet. The symptoms are often worst at night. Many people with diabetes have minor forms of neuropathy without knowing it, the problem only coming to light when a doctor tests for it.

The main problem for people with neuropathy is that, because they can't feel things going wrong with a foot, for example, they may not take the usual precautions against small injuries, infections or burns. I've known a man who lost half of his foot when a coal from the fire fell upon it. He was only made aware of his injury when he smelled the burning flesh.

That was an extreme case. Much more common are neglected small sores that develop into ulcers, and athlete's foot that doesn't itch and so spreads until it is almost impossible to cure.

Neuropathic ulcers are 'punched out', open wounds under the pressure pads below the foot, the heel, or on the tips or 'knuckles' of the toes. They need to be treated by specialists in foot care to clean them out, but also to treat any infection and to take off the pressure that caused the ulcer.

If you have neuropathy, you must take special care of your feet. You must keep them clean and dry, examine them for any sores, bruises or infection several times a week, and regularly see the chiropodist (podiatrist) associated with your diabetes team. If you have any physical problems, like poor eyesight or muscle weakness or shaking, don't cut your own toenails: you need a professional to do this.

It can't be repeated too often that the best way to control neuropathy, as with retinopathy and nephropathy, is to keep your blood glucose levels as close to normal as possible. It isn't easy to ease the nerve symptoms once they have started, but some people find that daily doses of 'tricyclic' drugs, more commonly used to treat depression, or the anti-epilepsy drug carbamazepine (Tegretol), help to reduce pain and the pins and needles. These drugs do not appear to improve the numbness, however, so they are no substitute for meticulous foot care.

Chapter Fifteen

'Macrovascular' Complications

All through this book I have been harping on about heart attacks and strokes. They are what doctors define as the 'macrovascular' complications of diabetes.

Why they should particularly affect people with either type of diabetes is now quite clear. The constant contact of the artery walls with too much glucose, too much of the wrong types of fat, excessively high blood pressure and, in smokers, nicotine, carbon monoxide and chemicals from tars, all combine to accelerate the process that happens to everyone through life – atherosclerosis.

Atherosclerosis

Even in apparently healthy people, the process of atherosclerosis starts early in life, building up irregular and rough deposits of cholesterol- and triglyceride-laden fats in the lining of arteries throughout the body. Post-mortem examinations of young American soldiers killed in the Korean war showed that they all had the beginnings of atherosclerosis, even those as young as 18. There were streaks of fatty deposits in their coronary and brain arteries. As these streaks change and increase in size and number, they form the basis of 'plaques', raised and roughened areas of weakness in the artery wall. Eventually, at one of these weak spots a clot forms to block the vessel, or it splits, so that it bleeds into the surrounding tissues. If these incidents occur in the coronary artery they cause heart attacks. In the brain they cause strokes.

Atherosclerosis is universal in modern humans, but it is accelerated in diabetes. Age for age, people with diabetes have more plaques, which affect more arteries, and which are at a more advanced stage, than people without it. This not only explains why people with diabetes have more heart attacks and strokes than others, but also why they need amputations. The atheromatous process spreads into the arteries of the legs and feet, too, blocking off the circulation to them. This leads to poor circulation, which if not controlled and improved, ends as gangrene and the inevitability of amputation.

As we all get older, our risks of having a heart attack or stroke increase, decade by decade, from 40 onwards, but the upward slope of the increase is much steeper for people with diabetes than for people without the disease.

For women with diabetes the story is even worse. In the non-diabetic population, atherosclerosis is less severe in women than in men of the same age. A rough approximation is that women have a 10-year advantage in the progression of their atherosclerosis over men, so that women of 60 have the same risk of heart attack and stroke as men of 50.

This is not the case for women with diabetes. Their diabetes seems to cancel out their natural advantage over men, a protection thought to be provided by their sex hormones throughout middle age. In fact, middle-aged women with diabetes are at higher risk of heart attacks and strokes than men of the same age who do not have diabetes.

We know very well the causes of the extra risks of heart attack and stroke: cigarette smoking, obesity, high blood pressure, high blood cholesterol levels, poor control of diabetes, and lack of exercise with a sedentary lifestyle. Tackle all of these together in the way this book has described, and you will hugely reduce your risk of all the macrovascular complications of your diabetes.

Peripheral Vascular Disease – Foot Problems

An extra word is needed here on the peripheral circulation – the arteries to the feet. Whether or not you have diabetic neuropathy (see Chapter Fourteen), if you have diabetes you are at high risk of having peripheral vascular disease (atherosclerosis of the arteries in the legs). This shows itself in pain in the legs on walking any distance, and in long-standing ulcers and infections that don't respond well or quickly to the usual treatments. Foot problems due to peripheral vascular disease account for a quarter of the admissions to hospital of all people with diabetes.

Your doctor and diabetes nurse will know something about your circulation from feeling the pulses in your groin, behind the knees, at your ankles and on the top of your feet. They can confirm suspicions of peripheral vascular disease by ultrasound and X-ray tests ('angiography') of the circulation in your legs. If you are found to have it, you absolutely MUST stop smoking and must even avoid other people's smoke. Smoking is the biggest factor in promoting peripheral vascular disease. If you continue with it, you will certainly lose your legs, and probably your life, as it strongly correlates with fatal heart attacks in amputees.

Diabetic peripheral vascular disease, unsurprisingly, is treated by maintaining good glucose control, lowering blood pressure, attending to cholesterol levels and, as far as possible, improving exercise levels. This may be difficult if walking is painful for you, but it is best to try to improve your walking distance gradually with a planned exercise programme.

Chapter Sixteen

Less Common Problems

The most common form of diabetic neuropathy was described in Chapter Fourteen (see pages 110-111). Other neuropathies are less common, but deserve mention.

Mononeuritis

Mononeuritis is a condition affecting a single nerve. This can be the nerve to one of the eye muscles, so that you develop a squint. Another common site is the nerve to the shoulder or buttocks and thighs, so that the muscles are first very painful, then become weak and waste away. This is called 'neuralgic amyotrophy'. It can leave the shoulder or the buttock and thigh weakened and even paralysed for several months, but it usually goes away, quite suddenly, up to 18 months or two years later.

Autonomic Neuropathy

In autonomic neuropathy the nerves affected are those controlling regulation of blood pressure, the digestion and the bladder. People with it tend to faint when they stand up after lying down or being seated for a while ('postural hypotension') because of a sudden drop in blood pressure. Or they have bouts of diarrhoea or an inability to pass urine when they wish to. They may sweat profusely after meals.

Autonomic neuropathy has no specific treatment except for better glucose control, so if you have it, you usually have to live with it. But if you ever have to have an operation you must tell the anaesthetist beforehand, as it can lead to complications with the anaesthetic.

Impotence/Loss of Enjoyment in Sex

Probably the best-known and most worrying of the neuropathies that affect people with diabetes is impotence in men and loss of previous enjoyment in love-making (not loss of libido, necessarily) in women. If this is one of your problems, please tell your diabetes team about it: most people keep it secret, which is a shame because it is certainly treatable.

The problem in both sexes seems to be a mixture of neuropathy and peripheral vascular disease affecting the nerves and circulation to the genital organs. Impotence is a very obvious failure in men. Only in the last few years, however, has it been understood that the clitoris is a much larger organ in women than it was thought. Bigger even than the erect penis, it extends up into the vagina and surrounds it in a tube of tissue that erects when filled with blood, just like the penis, when the woman is sexually excited.

The importance of this information (discovered by two female Australian anatomists in 2000) is that it explains why women, as well as men, with sexual problems due to neuropathy can derive great benefit from sildefanil (Viagra), the anti-impotence drug. In Britain, impotence associated with diabetes is an official indication for sildefanil. Many doctors are now finding it to be successful in women with the corresponding problem.

Chapter Seventeen

Diabetes in Pregnancy

Mary, one of the people with diabetes described in Chapter Two (page 15), had 'gestational diabetes'. Diabetes during pregnancy is not true diabetes. In Mary's case, the only problem was the finding of glucose in her urine, and it did not lead to overt diabetes. However, she was advised to follow a strict healthy eating and exercise regimen, mainly to prevent any complications during the pregnancy. She was then followed up for a year or two, to ensure that true diabetes did not develop afterwards. Her diagnosis of gestational diabetes remains in her medical records for future reference, as 40 per cent of women with gestational diabetes later develop diabetes.

However, what about the woman who already has diabetes who has become pregnant? Many women with Type 1 diabetes in particular face problems in pregnancy, including rapidly worsening kidney disease and eyesight.

They should therefore not undertake becoming pregnant lightly. They should weigh up the pros (usually the great desire to have a child) against the cons (substantial deterioration in their diabetes control and the possibility of permanent deterioration of their physical condition).

If you have diabetes and become pregnant, see your doctor immediately, so that you and your diabetes team can plan ahead. Don't wait the usual 8 weeks or so to sign up at the antenatal clinic. If you have Type 2 diabetes, for example, you may well have to go on insulin, as oral drugs are not given during pregnancy. An after-meal blood glucose level persistently above 8 mmol/L suggests you need to go on insulin.

You must expect at some time in the pregnancy for your diabetes control to go haywire, so expect to be admitted to hospital during the pregnancy to change your insulin dose or to deal with unexpected hyper or hypo attacks.

Don't, if you are pregnant, try to cope with all these problems yourself. You will have emergency phone numbers to ring, 24 hours a day, so use them if you have doubts.

When the baby is born, he or she is likely to be bigger than normal (often over 10 pounds), and less active than babies born to mothers who do not have diabetes. This is usual, and not a sign that the baby will have diabetes, but rather just the consequence of the extra glucose he or she has been exposed to in the womb. It does no long-term harm, and is usually coped with quite routinely by the staff caring for the new-born.

After the birth you will be faced with the question of whether to bottle-feed or breastfeed the baby. Choose the breast, by all means, but discuss the difference this will make to your blood glucose control with your diabetes team, and change your routine accordingly. Remember that while looking after a small child you cannot afford to have hypos or hypers, so you have an extra responsibility to keep your diabetes under good control.

Chapter Eighteen

Future Treatments

The future of diabetes treatment may lie with surgeons rather than with general practitioners. Already many people who have had serious, life-threatening forms of diabetes, whose kidneys have failed and for whom even the strictest control of blood glucose with insulin and diet have failed to prevent severe complications, are being helped by transplants.

In our practice we have been hugely encouraged by one young woman who was nearly blind and on daily dialysis for kidney failure. She was at considerable risk of heart attack and stroke. She received her pancreas and kidney transplant nearly three years ago, and is doing fantastically well, she no longer has diabetes. Her new pancreas and kidney are working beautifully and her anti-rejection drugs have so far kept complications at bay. Her vision has actually improved so much that she is able to drive her car again and look after her nine-year-old son.

Only a few centres of excellence in Britain can offer pancreatic/kidney transplants at the time of writing (April, 2001), but as more surgeons are trained, these centres will be more widespread. Whole pancreases may not be needed. Much research is going on into implanting 'bags' of pancreatic beta-cells into the abdomen, in which the membrane surrounding the cells allows in enough oxygen to keep them alive and functioning, but keep out the patient's white cells, which would initiate the process of rejection. If the techniques for growing beta-cells in the laboratory improve, we may see these implants being used very often in years to come.

Researchers are also well on their way to discovering how to convert 'stem cells' (primitive cells which can be persuaded to grow into mature tissue cells by the addition of substances called growth factors) to beta-cells. The aim is to collect such stem cells from patients' own blood or bone marrow, convert them into beta-cells, grow them profusely in the laboratory, then implant them into the liver, where they will flourish naturally and produce insulin.

Stem cell research may be a little further off than the implants, but be sure that one day it will lead to practical treatment for diabetes. And be sure, too, that there will be techniques for diabetes that are not yet thought of. One, for example, may be to determine at birth who is going to develop either type of diabetes, and to immunize them against it.

We are only at the beginning of a huge revolution in medicine. If this book is still in print 50 years from now, the chapters on treatment will look very different indeed.

Useful Addresses

All people with diabetes should be in regular contact with their local diabetes team. This team will comprise a minimum of a general practitioner, a dietician, a diabetes nurse, a chiropodist and an ophthalmologist – who are there for all the routine tasks described in this book – together with a diabetes specialist for the times when extra help is needed.

This team will be a great source of information on helpful local organizations who can provide support when it is needed. The most important organization for British people with diabetes is Diabetes UK (formerly the British Diabetic Association), to which all people with diabetes and their families should belong. Diabetes UK combines continuing research with educational programmes for everyone with diabetes and their families, and has local groups to provide the personal touch.

Diabetes UK

10 Queen Anne Street
London W1M 0BD
Tel: 0207 323 1531

Diabetes UK Scotland

140 Sauchiehall Street
Glasgow G2 3DH
Tel: 0141 332 2700

Glossary

Arteries Blood vessels taking blood from the heart to the rest of the body and to the lungs.

Auto-immune disease A state in which the body's immune system mistakes normal tissues as 'foreign' (i.e. like a virus or cancer cell), and starts to destroy them. Type 1 diabetes is an auto-immune disease, in which the immune system destroys the ability of the pancreas to produce insulin. This may also happen in some cases of Type 2 diabetes.

Beta-cells The cells in the pancreas that produce insulin.

Capillaries The smallest blood vessels, between the arteries and veins, through the walls of which glucose and oxygen must pass to provide the tissues with fuel and energy.

Cholesterol A form of fat in the blood. Divided into HDL (high-density lipoprotein) and LDL (low-density lipoprotein), the former removing fats from blood vessel walls, the latter depositing fat into them. So a high HDL cholesterol and a low LDL cholesterol are aimed for.

Glucagon A hormone with actions opposite to those of insulin. Used to treat insulin overdose.

Glycaemia The amount of glucose in the blood.

Glycaemic index The speed with which, and the height to which, a particular food will raise the blood glucose after being swallowed. People with diabetes should avoid foods with a high glycaemic index unless they are prepared to counter the rise in blood glucose with insulin, exercise or both.

Glycogen The form in which the body stores glucose. Only the liver and the muscles can store glycogen. It is quickly turned into glucose when needed, by the action of insulin.

HbA1c, also known as glycosylated haemoglobin. The percentage of red blood cells that are coated with glucose. The higher the HbA1c, the poorer the diabetes control has been in the previous three to four months.

Hyperglycaemia Too much glucose in the blood.

Hypoglycaemia Too little glucose in the blood.

Hypoglycaemic agents Drugs that lower blood glucose levels.

Insulin The substance made by the pancreas that drives glucose from the liver into the blood and from the blood into the tissues. By doing so, insulin provides all the vital organs with their supply of 'fuel'.

Ketones Substances appearing in the breath and urine when diabetes is out of control, and the body has to rely on fats (rather than glucose) for energy.

Ketosis (keto-acidosis) A state in which diabetes control is so poor that the ketones in the blood are causing physical and mental symptoms. Uncorrected, it may lead to coma.

Lipids Fats. The important ones for people with diabetes are cholesterol and triglycerides. High levels of these in the blood raise the risk of heart attacks and strokes.

Lipo-atrophy Loss of fatty tissue under the skin due to repeated insulin injections.

Lipohypertrophy Overgrowth of tissues under the skin in response to repeated insulin injections.

Metabolic syndrome A condition that combines high blood pressure, high cholesterol levels, Type 2 diabetes and obesity. Common in older people, all aspects of metabolic syndrome need to be treated, not just the diabetes.

Microalbuminuria Tiny amounts of protein in the urine predicting later kidney disease.

Nephropathy Signs of kidney problems.

Neuropathy Signs of problems affecting the nerves to the limbs and internal organs, such as the bladder and sex organs.

Pancreas The organ that produces insulin.

Proteinuria Sign of kidney damage due to diabetes or to kidney infections.

Retinopathy Signs of blood vessel problems in the eyes.

Syndrome X A version of metabolic syndrome that can pre-date the onset of diabetes.

Triglycerides A form of fat in the blood (see cholesterol) that is often raised in poorly controlled diabetes. The aim is to lower them to normal levels.

UKPDS United Kingdom Prospective Diabetes Study

Veins The blood vessels carrying blood from the rest of the body and from the lungs to the heart.

References

Chapter Eight
1 Amos, A F, McCarty, D J, Zimmet, P, 'The rising global burden of diabetes and its complications: estimates and projections to the year 2010', *Diabetic Medicine* 14, supp. 5 (1997): 1-895
2 Tuomi, T, Groop, L C, Zimmit, P *et al.*, 'Antibodies to glutamic acid decarboxylase reveal latent autoimmune diabetes mellitus in adults with a non-insulin-dependent onset of disease', *Diabetes* 42 (1993): 159-62

Index

Acarbose 46, 88, 90, 91, 92
Adolescence 23
Alcohol 17, 27, 37, 47, 49, 50, 51, 82, 85, 107
Alpha-glucosidase inhibitors 87
American Diabetes Association 72
Artificial sweeteners 44
Atherosclerosis 113, 114
Atrophy 58
Biguanides 87
Body mass index 49
Cataract 70, 110
Cholesterol 18, 46-48, 75-77, 80, 81, 93, 97, 103,
                                                                105, 106, 113-115
Clitoris 118
Cohen, Dr Matthew 82
Coma 20, 28, 32, 34, 75
Complications 9, 13, 20, 23, 24, 26, 58, 60, 67, 78-80,
                             87, 103, 109-111, 113, 114, 117, 119, 121, 126
Diabetes UK 123
Diarrhoea 35, 90, 91, 117
Diet 9, 15-17, 25-27, 41-44, 46, 77, 78, 121
Feet 26, 85, 91, 111-114
Fish 47, 48
'Gestational diabetes' 16, 119
Glucagon 38, 89, 90
Glycogen 12, 33, 69, 90
Glycosuria 18, 59
Gray, Alastair 80
Haemoglobin 24
HbA1c 24-26, 28, 29, 31, 54, 60, 77, 78, 84, 91, 94, 110
Hyperglycaemia 11, 31-33, 45, 77
Hypo 11, 20, 23, 28, 29, 31, 37-39, 45, 51, 53, 55, 56,
                                        62, 75, 82, 89, 90, 119, 120
Hypoglycaemic 11, 28, 31, 36, 37, 79, 82, 84, 87, 88, 93
Impotence 51, 117, 118
Insulin pens 57
Insulin resistance 18, 68, 70, 72, 88, 91
Keen, Professor Harry 75

Ketoacidosis 34, 35, 75
Ketones 12, 28, 32-34, 36
Ketosis.. 28, 29, 33
Lactic acidosis 31
Lipohypertrophy...57, 58
Medicalert 33, 38
Metabolic syndrome 73, 76, 81, 93, 104
Microalbuminuria....................26, 75, 76, 81, 104, 111
Nauraun islanders 67
Nephropathy 109, 110, 112
Neuropathy 26, 51, 60, 84, 85, 109-112, 114, 117, 118
Oral glucose tolerance test 16, 72
Orgogozo, Professor Jean-Marc...................................... 49
Pancreas........................... 9, 11, 17, 19, 53, 61, 68, 69,
                                                           88, 91, 92, 121
Pancreatitis.. 17, 19
Pima Indians 67, 68
Pregnancy 16, 27, 119
Reaven, Dr G M 68, 75, 76
Retinopathy... 26, 109, 110, 112
Rosiglitazone 92
Sildefanil 118
Smoking 5, 62, 63, 75, 77, 80, 85, 87, 97-102, 114
Statin...18, 106
Redgrave, Sir Steven 4, 12, 62
Sulphonylureas 78, 79, 87-92, 106
Syndrome X 18, 76
Tattersall, Professor Robert 20
Teenage 5, 23, 27, 69, 70
Thrush.. 14, 15, 70, 71
United Kingdom Prospective
  Diabetes Study (UKPDS) 73, 75-80, 93, 103, 104
World Health Organisation... 72
Zimmet Professor Paul 70, 82, 126